Curbside Consultation
in IBD

49 Clinical Questions

CURBSIDE CONSULTATION IN GASTROENTEROLOGY
SERIES

SERIES EDITOR, FRANCIS A. FARRAYE, MD, MSc, FACG, FASGE

Curbside Consultation

in IBD

49 Clinical Questions

EDITED BY

David T. Rubin, MD, FACG, AGAF
Co-Director, Inflammatory Bowel Disease Center
Program Director, Fellowship in Gastroenterology,
Hepatology and Nutrition
University of Chicago Medical Center
Chicago, IL

Sonia Friedman, MD
Associate Physician, Brigham and Women's Hospital
Gastroenterology Division ASBII
Boston, MA

Francis A. Farraye, MD, MSc, FACG, FASGE
Clinical Director, Section of Gastroenterology
Boston Medical Center
Boston, MA

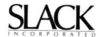
SLACK
INCORPORATED

www.slackbooks.com

ISBN: 978-1-55642-856-2

Published by: SLACK Incorporated
                   6900 Grove Road
                   Thorofare, NJ 08086 USA
                   Telephone: 856-848-1000
                   Fax: 856-848-6091
                   www.slackbooks.com

Contact SLACK Incorporated for more information about other books in this field or about the availability of our books from distributors outside the United States.

Library of Congress Cataloging-in-Publication Data

Curbside consultation in IBD : 49 clinical questions / edited by David T. Rubin, Sonia Friedman, Francis A. Farraye.
     p. ; cm. -- (Curbside consultation in gastroenterology)
  Includes bibliographical references and index.
  ISBN 978-1-55642-856-2 (alk. paper)
  1. Inflammatory bowel diseases. I. Rubin, David T., 1968- II. Friedman, Sonia. III. Farraye, Francis A. IV. Series: Curbside consultation in gastroenterology.
  [DNLM: 1. Inflammatory Bowel Diseases. WI 420 C975 2009]
  RC862.I53C867 2009
  616.3′44--dc22
                         2008054824

Printed in the United States of America.

Last digit is print number: 10   9   8   7   6   5   4   3   2   1

Dedication

This book is dedicated to my wife Rebecca, my sons Danny and Michael, and to all of the patients who inspire me to find better answers.
-*David T. Rubin, MD, FACG, AGAF*

This book is dedicated to my supportive and loving husband, Jerry, and to my wonderful children, Sam and Angela. It is also dedicated to my parents, who encouraged me daily to work my hardest and who are always there for me when I need them.
-*Sonia Friedman, MD*

This book is dedicated to my loving and devoted family: my wife, Renee M. Remily, MD; my children, Jennifer and Alexis Farraye; and to my parents, who taught me that perseverance and commitment can result in great accomplishments.
-*Francis A. Farraye, MD, MSc, FACG, FASGE*

Contents

Acknowledgments

We are very grateful to our authors who selflessly shared their experience and evidence-based knowledge with us in highly readable and relevant chapters. We remain grateful and humbled by your friendship and collegiality.

We are also indebted to the support, guidance, and patience of the terrific team at SLACK Incorporated, including Carrie Kotlar, Senior Acquisitions Editor, and Debra Toulson, Managing Editor.

Finally, we are thankful to you, the reader, who has identified the exciting field of inflammatory bowel disease as one in which you seek to learn more and remain current. We appreciate your efforts and know your patients will as well.

About the Editors

David T. Rubin, MD, FACG, AGAF is an Associate Professor of Medicine, the Program Director for the Fellowship in Gastroenterology, Hepatology, and Nutrition, and the Co-Director of the Inflammatory Bowel Disease Center at the University of Chicago Medical Center in Chicago, IL. He is an Associate Faculty Member of the University of Chicago MacLean Center for Clinical Medical Ethics, and an investigator in the Cancer Research Center of the University of Chicago.

Dr. Rubin earned his doctor of medicine degree with honors from the University of Chicago Pritzker School of Medicine. He completed his residency in internal medicine and both of his fellowships in gastroenterology and clinical medical ethics at the University of Chicago, where he served as Chief Resident and Chief Fellow.

Dr. Rubin is a member of the American Gastroenterology Association (AGA), previously serving on the Ethics Committee and currently serving on the Subcommittee for Training and the Public Affairs and Advocacy Committee. He is a Fellow of the American College of Gastroenterology (ACG), serving on the Professional Issues and Publications Committee. He is also a member of the Crohn's and Colitis Foundation of America (CCFA) and has chaired the CCFA Illinois Educational Program from 2005 to 2008. He also served as Chair of Professional Education for CCFA nationally, and directed the national fellowship and preceptorship programs from 2005-2008.

An avid researcher, Dr. Rubin's interests include clinical outcomes of inflammatory bowel disease (IBD), colon cancer screening and prevention, teaching medicine, and clinical medical ethics. He is currently the principal investigator for several research projects and clinical trials involving wireless capsule endoscopy in IBD, measures of inflammation and cancer risk, and novel technologies for disease monitoring. Dr. Rubin has contributed numerous peer-reviewed publications, book chapters, review articles, and abstracts to the medical literature, including a previous handbook for the hospitalized IBD patient.

Sonia Friedman, MD is an Assistant Professor of Medicine at Harvard Medical School in Boston, MA, and an Associate Physician at Brigham and Women's Hospital, also in Boston. Dr. Friedman completed her undergraduate degree in biology at Stanford University in Palo Alto, CA, and her medical degree at Yale University School of Medicine in New Haven, CT. She did her medical internship and residency at the University of Pennsylvania in Philadelphia, PA, and her gastroenterology fellowship at Mount Sinai Medical Center in New York, NY. She specialized in IBD during her fellowship and now has a large IBD practice in the gastroenterology division of Brigham and Women's Hospital. She has been at Brigham and Women's for the past 9 years, and is Director of IBD Clinical Research.

Dr. Friedman's research interests include colon cancer in Crohn's disease (CD), patient adherence to surveillance colonoscopy and to IBD medications, and IBD and pregnancy. Her clinical interests are the care of patients with CD and ulcerative colitis (UC). She specializes in the management of dysplasia and cancer in IBD, and pregnancy and IBD.

Dr. Friedman is a frequent speaker and invited regional and national lecturer on the management of IBD. She has authored or coauthored peer-reviewed papers on cancer in CD, management of polyps and cancer in IBD, medical management of IBD, and pregnancy and IBD. She has written review articles and chapters on various aspects of IBD, including the IBD chapter in *Harrison's Principles of Internal Medicine*. Her publications include original articles, reviews, or chapters in *Gastroenterology*, *Clinical Gastroenterology and Hepatology*, *American Journal of Gastroenterology*, *Inflammatory Bowel Diseases*, and *Gastroenterology Clinics of North America*. She is section editor for *Inflammatory Bowel Diseases*, and is a reviewer for *Gastroenterology*, *Clinical Gastroenterology and Hepatology*, and *American Journal of Gastroenterology*.

Dr. Friedman is chair-elect of the CCFA New England Chapter Medical Advisory Committee, and is co-chair of their annual patient symposium. She is a Fellow of the ACG and has served on the CCFA Professional Education Committee. She has been elected as "Best Up-and-Coming Gastroenterologist in Boston" in 2004, and was also listed as "Best of Boston" in *Boston Magazine* in 2007. Both honors are based upon peer review.

Francis A. Farraye, MD, MSc, FACG, FASGE is a Professor of Medicine at the Boston University School of Medicine in Boston, MA. He is also Clinical Director in the Section of Gastroenterology and Co-Director of the Center for Digestive Disorders at Boston Medical Center. After graduating from the State University of New York (SUNY) at Stony Brook, Dr. Farraye earned his medical doctorate from Albert Einstein College of Medicine in New York, NY, and his master's degree in Epidemiology from the Harvard School of Public Health in Boston, MA. He completed an internal medicine residency and gastroenterology fellowship at the Beth Israel Hospital in Boston.

Dr. Farraye's clinical interests are in the care of patients with IBD, the management of colon polyps and colorectal cancer, as well endoscopy in patients after bariatric surgery. He is studying Vitamin D absorption in patients with IBD, the management and diagnosis of dysplasia and cancer in patients with IBD, and predictors of pouchitis after ileal pouch-anal anastomosis (IPAA). In the area of colorectal cancer, he is examining the role of hyperplastic polyps as an alternative pathway in the development of colorectal cancer.

A frequent speaker and invited lecturer on topics on the diagnosis and management of IBD, Dr. Farraye has authored or coauthored over 150 original scientific manuscripts, chapters, reviews, and abstracts. His work has been published in the *American Journal of Gastroenterology*, *Gastroenterology*, *Alimentary Pharmacology and Therapeutics*, *Gastrointestinal Endoscopy*, *Annals of Internal Medicine*, and *JAMA*, among others. He is a coeditor for the text *Bariatric Surgery: A Primer for your Medical Practice*, and an associate editor for *Therapy for Digestive Disorders*. He recently edited an issue of *Gastroenterology Clinics of North America* on dysplasia and cancer in IBD. He is the series editor for the *Curbside Consultations in Gastroenterology* series.

Dr. Farraye is a Fellow of the American College of Physicians, American Society of Gastrointestinal Endoscopy, and the ACG. Nationally, he serves as Chair of the Board of Governors and a member of the Board of Trustees in the ACG. He has served as the AGA representative on the National Colorectal Cancer Round Table as Co-Chair of the

Standards Committee and as Chair of the Lower Gastrointestinal Disorders Section of the Annual Scientific Program Committee of the ASGE. He is a member of the ASGE Technology Committee, CCFA Professional Education Committee, and the Chapter Medical Advisory Committee for the New England CCFA, where he is a past chairman. The New England CCFA named Dr. Farraye "Humanitarian of the Year" in 2003.

Contributing Authors

Maria T. Abreu, MD (Question 48)
Professor of Medicine
Chief, Division of Gastroenterology
University of Miami Miller School of
    Medicine
Miami, FL

Charles N. Bernstein, MD (Question 43)
Professor of Medicine
Head, Section of Gastroenterology
Director, University of Manitoba IBD
    Clinical and Research Center
Winnipeg, Manitoba, Canada

David G. Binion, MD (Question 42)
Co-Director, Inflammatory Bowel Disease
    Center
Director, Translational Inflammatory
    Bowel Disease Research
Visiting Professor of Medicine
Division of Gastroenterology, Hepatology
    and Nutrition
University of Pittsburgh School of
    Medicine
Pittsburgh, PA

Wojciech Blonski, MD, PhD (Question 34)
Division of Gastroenterology
University of Pennsylvania
Philadelphia, PA
Department of Gastroenterology and
    Hepatology
Medical University
Wroclaw, Poland

*Robert Burakoff, MD, MPH, FACG, FACP
    (Question 49)*
Clinical Chief, Division of
    Gastroenterology
Director, Center for Digestive Health
Brigham and Women's Hospital
Associate Professor of Medicine
Harvard Medical School
Boston, MA

Adam S. Cheifetz, MD (Question 46)
Assistant Professor of Medicine
Harvard Medical School
Clinical Director, Center for Inflammatory
    Bowel Disease
Beth Israel Deaconess Medical Center
Boston, MA

*Russell D. Cohen, MD, FACG, AGAF
    (Questions 36, 39)*
Associate Professor of Medicine
Co-Director, Inflammatory Bowel Disease
    Center
University of Chicago Medical Center
Chicago, IL

Carmen Cuffari, MD (Question 37)
Division of Pediatric GI
Johns Hopkins Hospital
Baltimore, MD

Kleanthis Dendrinos, MD (Questions 1, 18)
Fellow in Gastroenterology
Boston University Medical Center
Boston, MA

Marla C. Dubinsky, MD (Questions 20, 27)
Director, Pediatric IBD Center
Cedars-Sinai Medical Center
Los Angeles, CA

Sarah N. Flier, MD (Question 46)
Fellow in Gastroenterology
Beth Israel Deaconess Medical Center
Boston, MA

*Stephen B. Hanauer, MD, FACG, AGAF
    (Questions 3, 4)*
Professor of Medicine and Clinical
    Pharmacology
Chief, Section of Gastroenterology,
    Hepatology and Nutrition
University of Chicago Medical Center
Chicago, IL

Kim L. Isaacs, MD, PhD, AGAF (Question 26)
Professor of Medicine
Division of Gastroenterology and
    Hepatology
University of North Carolina
Chapel Hill, NC

*Sunanda Kane, MD, MSPH, FACG, FACP,
    AGAF (Question 22)*
Associate Professor of Medicine
Miles and Shirley Fiterman Division of
    Gastroenterology and Hepatology
Mayo Clinic College of Medicine
Rochester, MN

*Marshall M. Kaplan, MD, MACP (Question
    28)*
Chief Emeritus, Division of
    Gastroenterology
Tufts Medical Center
Professor of Medicine
Tufts University School of Medicine
Boston, MA

Asher Kornbluth, MD (Question 29)
Clinical Professor of Medicine
The Dr. Henry D. Janowitz Division of
    Gastroenterology
Department of Medicine
Mount Sinai Medical Center
New York, NY

Joshua R. Korzenik, MD (Question 40)
Co-Director, Crohn's and Colitis Center
Massachusetts General Hospital
Boston, MA

David Kotlyar, BS (Question 34)
University of Pennsylvania School of
    Medicine
Philadelphia, PA

Bret A. Lashner, MD (Question 17)
Professor of Medicine
Director, Center for Inflammatory Bowel
    Disease
Cleveland Clinic
Cleveland, OH

Mark Lazarev, MD (Question 5)
Present-Levison Inflammatory Bowel
    Disease Fellow
Mount Sinai Medical Center
New York, NY

*Jonathan A. Leighton, MD, FACG, AGAF
    (Question 24)*
Professor of Medicine
Chair, Division of Gastroenterology and
    Hepatology
Mayo Clinic
Scottsdale, AZ

L. Campbell Levy, MD (Question 7)
Assistant Professor of Medicine
Dartmouth Medical School
Section of Gastroenterology and
    Hepatology
Dartmouth-Hitchcock Medical Center
Lebanon, NH

*James D. Lewis, MD, MSCE, AGAF
    (Question 38)*
Associate Professor of Medicine and
    Epidemiology
Senior Scholar in the Center for Clinical
    Epidemiology and Biostatistics
Associate Director, Center for
    Inflammatory Bowel Disease
University of Pennsylvania
Philadelphia, PA

Gary R. Lichtenstein, MD (Question 34)
Professor of Medicine
Director, Center for Inflammatory Bowel
    Diseases
Divison of Gastroenterology
Department of Internal Medicine
Hospital of the University of Pennsylvania
Philadelphia, PA

Edward V. Loftus, Jr., MD (Question 23)
Professor of Medicine
Chair, Inflammatory Bowel Disease
    Interest Group
Miles and Shirley Fiterman Center for
    Digestive Diseases
Mayo Clinic
Rochester, MN

Uma Mahadevan-Velayos, MD (Question 21)
Associate Professor of Medicine
Director, Clinical Research
UCSF Center for Colitis and Crohn's
 Disease
San Francisco, CA

Juan L. Mendoza, MD, PhD (Question 48)
Inflammatory Bowel Disease Center
Mount Sinai School of Medicine
New York, NY

Seamus J. Murphy, PhD, MRCP (Question 29)
Consultant Gastroenterologist
Southern Health and Social Care Trust
Craigavon Area Hospital
Portadown, Craigavon
County Armagh, Northern Ireland

Remo Panaccione, MD, FRCPC (Questions 6, 47)
Director, Inflammatory Bowel Disease
 Clinic
Director, Gastroenterology Training
 Program
Associate Professor of Medicine
University of Calgary
Calgary, Alberta, Canada

Darrell S. Pardi, MD, FACG, AGAF (Question 31)
Associate Professor of Medicine
Division of Gastroenterology and
 Hepatology
Mayo Clinic College of Medicine
Rochester, MN

Daniel H. Present, MD, MACG (Question 10)
Clinical Professor of Medicine
Mount Sinai School of Medicine
New York, NY

Abrar Qureshi, MD, MPH (Question 45)
Assistant Professor of Dermatology
Harvard Medical School
Department of Dermatology
Brigham and Women's Hospital
Boston, MA

Miguel Regueiro, MD (Question 5)
Associate Professor of Medicine
Co-Director, Inflammatory Bowel Disease
 Center
Director, Gastroenterology, Hepatology
 and Nutrition Fellowship
UPMC-PUH
Pittsburgh, PA

Rene Rivera, MD (Question 30)
Clinical Associate
Digestive Disease Institute
Nutrition Support Team
Cleveland Clinic
Cleveland, OH

Paul Rutgeerts, MD, PhD, FRCP (Questions 8, 33)
Department of Gastroenterology
University Hospital Gasthuisberg
Belgium

David A. Schwartz, MD (Question 41)
Director, Inflammatory Bowel Disease
 Center
Associate Professor of Medicine
Vanderbilt University Medical Center
Nashville, TN

Douglas L. Seidner, MD, FACG (Question 30)
Associate Professor of Medicine
Division of Gastroenterology, Hepatology
 and Nutrition
Director, Vanderbilt Center for Human
 Nutrition
Vanderbilt University Medical Center
Nashville, TN

Bo Shen, MD, FACG (Question 25)
Digestive Disease Institute
The Cleveland Clinic Foundation
Cleveland, OH

Corey A. Siegel, MD (Question 7)
Assistant Professor of Medicine
Dartmouth Medical School
Director, Inflammatory Bowel Disease
   Center
Section of Gastroenterology and
   Hepatology
Dartmouth-Hitchcock Medical Center
Lebanon, NH

Miles Sparrow, MB, BS, FRACP (Question 9)
Consultant Gastroenterologist
Department of Gastroenterology
Box Hill and The Alfred Hospitals
Melbourne, Australia

*A. Hillary Steinhart, MD, MSc, FRCPC
   (Questions 11, 12)*
Head, Combined Division of
   Gastroenterology
Mount Sinai Hospital/University Health
   Network
Associate Professor of Medicine
University of Toronto
Toronto, Canada

Arun Swaminath, MD (Question 16)
Assistant Professor in Clinical Medicine
Department of Medicine
Division of Digestive and Liver Diseases
Columbia University Presbyterian
   Hospital
New York, NY

Linda Tang, MD (Question 43)
University of Manitoba IBD Clinical and
   Research Center
Winnipeg, Manitoba, Canada

William J. Tremaine, MD (Question 35)
Maxine and Jack Zarrow Professor of
   Medicine
Division of Gastroenterology and
   Hepatology
Mayo Clinic
Rochester, MN

Thomas A. Ullman, MD, FACG (Question 16)
The Dr. Henry D. Janowitz Division of
   Gastroenterology
Mount Sinai School of Medicine
New York, NY

Gert van Assche, MD, PhD (Questions 8, 33)
Department of Gastroenterology
University Hospital of Leuven
Belgium

*Séverine Vermeire, MD, PhD (Questions 8,
   33)*
Department of Gastroenterology
University Hospital of Leuven
Belgium

*Jerome D. Waye, MD, FACG, AGAF, FASGE
   (Question 32)*
Past President, American Society for
   Gastrointestinal Endoscopy
Past President, American College of
   Gastroenterology
President-Elect, World Organization of
   Digestive Endoscopy
Clinical Professor of Medicine
Mount Sinai Medical Center
New York, NY

Laura S. Winterfield, MD (Question 45)
Clinical Director, Pyoderma Gangrenosum
   Clinic
Department of Dermatology
Brigham and Women's Hospital
Boston, MA

Preface

Perhaps no other field in gastroenterology epitomizes the rapid advance of science and medicine, and clinician and patient efforts to keep up with these developments, than inflammatory bowel disease (IBD). In the last decade, the treatment options for both Crohn's disease (CD) and ulcerative colitis (UC) have expanded to include entirely new classes of compounds, as well as improvements to existing fundamental therapies. This book, *Curbside Consultation in IBD*, has been compiled in an effort to grapple with 49 of the most common and potentially perplexing issues facing clinicians in the management of patients with IBD. The format of a question followed by a concise clinically-based answer by nationally and internationally recognized experts in our field offers a broad range of health care providers instant access to insight and information, which will be most useful in their daily practice.

A challenge in the composition and editing of this text was not only identifying the most pressing questions and issues facing our specialty, but also identifying those experts who can provide a glimpse into the current and near-future care of patients in these areas. We are grateful to our colleagues and coauthors from around the world who offered their insight and shared their time with us for the completion of this unique book.

We hope you find this text to be an informative addition to your clinical tools. We welcome your suggestions regarding common questions that we failed to include, or difficult questions for which you have been unable to find an answer in the literature. We are hopeful that these questions will provide the foundation for the next edition of *Curbside Consultation in IBD*.

Foreword

Whenever we give a lecture, web-cast, or symposium on IBD, the audience sits attentively and waits to ask their specific questions related to the "nitty gritty" of treating individual patients. For the most part, the questions are quite predictable and require the extrapolation and experience to translate evidence from basic or translational research or clinical trials into clinical practice.

IBD is one field where, despite a growing evidence base, the heterogeneity of disease presentations, responses to treatment, and the need to individualize therapy require more than controlled clinical trial data to optimize diagnostic and therapeutic outcomes. Indeed, even with taking the best evidence for our most sensitive diagnostics or potent therapies, there remains a substantial gap in potential outcomes. Whether we're handling questions regarding diagnostic schema, prognostication, or treatment outcomes, evidence from basic and clinical research is far from perfect, or even sufficient, to dictate management from diagnosis through induction and maintenance therapy, let alone how to approach complications of disease and treatment.

In an attempt to complement and supplement published evidence on the diagnosis and management of IBD, the editors have assimilated a group of key opinion leaders who have been the authors of the published evidence and are respected and experienced clinicians who provide consultations regarding patients with inadequate responses, poor outcomes, or those who fall within the gray areas that research does not address.

Drs. Rubin, Friedman, and Farraye have assimilated the preponderance of these "frequently asked questions" into a practical compendium that, indeed, will be useful for *Curbside Consultations in IBD*, or in this case, bed- or clinic-side consultations.

Stephen B. Hanauer, MD, FACG, AGAF
Professor of Medicine and Clinical Pharmacology
Chief, Section of Gastroenterology, Hepatology and Nutrition
University of Chicago Medical Center

I Recently Did a Colonoscopy on a Patient With Rectal Bleeding. The Patient Had Inflammation in the Rectosigmoid and Also in the Cecal Area. Is This Crohn's Disease?

Kleanthis Dendrinos, MD and
Francis A. Farraye, MD, MSc, FACG, FASGE

Colonoscopy plays an essential role in the evaluation of patients with rectal bleeding. In patients found to have colitis on colonoscopy, the distribution and appearance of the inflammatory process and the presence of "skip" lesions can help the endoscopist distinguish ulcerative colitis (UC) from Crohn's disease (CD). Mucosal biopsies can confirm a diagnosis of chronic inflammatory bowel disease (IBD), exclude other causes of colitis, and differentiate between UC and CD. However, as there can be overlap in the endoscopic and histologic appearance of UC and CD, the clinician often relies on the presence or absence of terminal ileal and/or upper gastrointestinal (GI) involvement to help distinguish CD from UC. Increasingly, serological testing including anti-Saccharomyces cerevisiae (ASCA), anti-nuclear cytoplasmic antibodies (ANCA), outer membrane porin protein C (ompC), and CBir1 (flagellin) have been used to distinguish CD from UC. Although medical therapy is often similar for patients with either UC or Crohn's colitis, the long-term prognosis and surgical management vary considerably between these 2 disorders. Therefore, making the correct diagnosis is vital with regard to making management decisions.

The traditional teaching is that the inflammation in UC involves the rectum and progresses proximally in a continuous fashion.[1] In contrast, CD often spares the rectum and can have "skip lesions." Skip lesions are areas of uninvolved mucosa both endoscopically and microscopically interspersed between inflamed tissue in the GI tract. However, several exceptions to the traditional teaching for differentiating between these 2 phenotypes of IBD have been described in recent years. As they relate to the patient described above, these include the presence of periappendiceal inflammation in patients with left-sided UC, a patchy disease that develops in patients with UC as a result of medical therapy ("cecal patch"), and patchy disease that develops in patients with UC as a result of medical therapy (Figure 1-1).

Several studies have evaluated patchy cecal and periappendiceal inflammation in patients with limited left-sided UC. D'Haens originally described this phenomenon in 1997.[2] D'Haens et al coined the term "cecal patch" to describe a subset of UC patients with left-sided colitis associated with cecal inflammation and who also had endoscopic and histologic sparing of the transverse colon. In their prospective study, 20 consecutive patients with established left-sided UC were followed for approximately 9 years. Fifteen patients (75%) were found to have periappendiceal inflammation that was separated from distally inflamed segments of the colon by areas of uninvolved mucosa. None of the patients developed features of CD.

In another prospective endoscopic and biopsy study by Yang et al, appendiceal orifice inflammation (AOI), as determined concomitantly by endoscopy and histology, was seen in 26% of 94 patients who had UC that did not extend proximally to the hepatic flexure.[3] There was no statistically significant difference in the prevalence of appendiceal orifice involvement between previously medically treated and newly diagnosed cases of UC, and thus, these authors concluded that appendiceal involvement was not due to the effects of medical therapy. In 2002, Matsumoto et al examined 40 patients with distal UC (including 10 patients who were presenting with their initial flare of UC) and found periappendiceal involvement in 23 (57%) of them.[4] In 2004, Mutinga et al compared clinical and pathologic features, as well as the natural history of disease, in a cohort of 12 patients with left-sided UC combined with patchy right colonic inflammation to a control group of 35 patients with isolated left-sided UC who were followed for almost 9 years. They found no differences between the two groups with regard to the severity of the disease, the prevalence of extraintestinal manifestations, a family history of colitis, or gender distribution. The only statistically significant difference between the groups was age. The subject group with patchy right colonic inflammation was noted to be about 10 years older. None of the subjects with patchy right-sided disease had disease progression to pancolitis, development of high-grade dysplasia (HGD), or clinical or pathologic features consistent with CD.[5]

Apparent skip lesions in UC may also develop in patients with UC over time or as a result of medical therapy. Kim et al studied 32 UC subjects on medical therapy who underwent serial colonoscopies for a period of up to 13 years. Patchy disease, rectal sparing, or both were found on follow-up colonoscopy in 59% of the patients.[6] In a 1995 study, Bernstein et al prospectively examined 39 UC subjects on medical therapy, and described endoscopic evidence of discontinuous patchiness in 44% of them.[7] Odze et al performed a prospective randomized study and found that 64% of the patients treated with 5-aminosalicyclic acid (5-ASA) enemas showed reversion of previously inflamed rectal mucosa to a completely normal state (without chronic or active inflammation) in at least one of the patients' rectal biopsies. Patients treated with 5-ASA enemas also showed a statistically higher percentage of normal biopsies (36%) per patient compared with the placebo-treated group (12%).[8] These studies suggest that skip lesions, including rectal sparing and patchiness of disease, may occur over time in patients with UC, and may be associated with medical therapy.

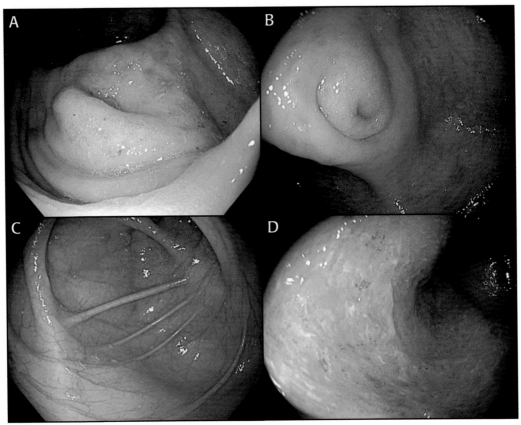

Figure 1-1. Periappendiceal inflammation (A, B). Normal transverse colon (C). Rectal inflammation (D).

In summary, UC patients with inflammation in the distal colon and cecum, as well as with endoscopic and histologic sparing of the remainder of the colon, should not be considered as having CD unless there are other features to suggest CD, such as deep fissuring ulcerations, evidence of fistula, or granulomas on histopathology. Assuming that there are no features to suggest small bowel involvement on imaging, the patient described above should be classified as having UC with a cecal patch.

References

1. Yantiss RK, Odze RD. Pitfalls in the interpretation of non-neoplastic mucosal biopsies in inflammatory bowel disease. *Am J Gastroenterol.* 2007;102(4):890-904.
2. D'Haens G, Geboes K, Peeters M, Baert F, Ectors N, Rutgeerts P. Patchy cecal inflammation associated with distal ulcerative colitis: a prospective endoscopic study. *Am J Gastroenterol.* 1997;92(8):1275-1279.
3. Yang SK, Jung HY, Kang GH, et al. Appendiceal orifice inflammation as a skip lesion in ulcerative colitis: an analysis in relation to medical therapy and disease extent. *Gastrointest Endosc.* 1999;49(6):743-747.
4. Matsumoto T, Nakamura S, Shimizu M, et al. Significance of appendiceal involvement in patients with ulcerative colitis. *Gastrointest Endosc.* 2002;55(2):180-185.
5. Mutinga ML, Odze RD, Wang HH, et al. The clinical significance of right-sided colonic inflammation in patients with left-sided chronic ulcerative colitis. *Inflamm Bowel Dis.* 2004;10(3):215-219.
6. Kim B, Barnett JL, Kleer CG, Appelman HD. Patchiness in treated ulcerative colitis. *Am J Gastroenterol.* 1999;94(11):3258-3262.

7. Bernstein CN, Shanahan F, Anton PA, Weinstein WM. Patchiness of mucosal inflammation in treated ulcerative colitis: a prospective study. *Gastrointest Endosc.* 1995;42(3):232-237.
8. Odze R, Antonioli D, Peppercorn M, Goldman H. Effect of topical 5-aminosalicylic acid (5-ASA) therapy on rectal mucosal biopsy morphology in chronic ulcerative colitis. *Am J Surg Pathol.* 1993;17(9):869-875.

WHEN IS IT APPROPRIATE TO SWITCH TO ANOTHER BIOLOGIC THERAPY?

David T. Rubin, MD, FACG, AGAF and Sonia Friedman, MD

Biologic therapy is often reserved for moderately to severely ill patients with Crohn's disease (CD) who have failed other therapies. Patients who respond to biologic therapies enjoy an improvement in clinical symptoms, a better quality of life, fewer surgeries and hospitalizations, and less disability, fatigue, and depression. The first biologic therapy approved for CD was infliximab, a chimeric immunoglobulin G1 (IgG1) antibody against tumor necrosis factor alpha (TNF-α), which is now also approved for the treatment of moderately to severely active ulcerative colitis (UC). Subsequently, the fully human adalimumab and humanized certolizumab pegol have been approved as injectable anti-TNF-α therapies for the treatment of moderately to severely active CD. An additional biologic therapy, natalizumab, an IgG4 antibody against the α4 subunit of α4beta1 (β1) and α4β7 on leukocytes, was approved as monotherapy for treatment of moderately to severely active CD patients failing or intolerant to TNF-α therapy. Natalizumab prevents recruitment of leukocytes to the area of disease and is a mechanism unique from the anti-TNF-α therapies.

As proteins that are infused or injected into patients, all of the biologic therapies have the potential to generate an immune response, and this immunogenicity may be associated with reactions to the drug and loss of response. Although this has best been described with infliximab, it likely occurs with all 4 available biologic therapies, regardless of how "humanized" they are. A number of strategies for minimization of immunogenicity have been described and recommended, including loading doses of the therapy to "tolerize" the immune system to them, committing to maintenance therapy, and using concomitant immunomodulator therapy. It has been shown that the most effective way to decrease antibody formation is by committing to maintenance therapy, though concomitant immunomodulators only reduce antibody formation by a smaller amount (about 4% to 10%). More importantly, the use of concomitant immunomodulatory therapy has largely fallen out of favor and is no longer recommended due to the emergence of a series of patients with hepatosplenic T-cell lymphoma (HSTCL), which is rare and usually lethal, as well as the increased understanding that concomitant therapy with immunosuppressives may increase the likelihood of serious or opportunistic infections.[1,2] In addition, review of subsets from all of the pivotal trials in infliximab, adalimumab, certolizumab pegol, and natalizumab have failed to demonstrate an efficacy benefit in response or maintenance, despite whether the patient was on immunomodulators or not on them. A subsequent study of withdrawal of the immunomodulatory therapy in patients in stable remission with infliximab failed to demonstrate an increased loss of response to therapy compared to the patients who remained on concomitant therapy.[3]

Despite best efforts, though, loss of response to a therapy is a common problem, and although it has been most described with infliximab, similar observations have been made with the other biologic therapies. Only one-third of patients who initially respond to infliximab, adalimumab, or certolizumab pegol therapy will be in remission after 1 year of treatment. How does one assess patients who have lost response, and when should they be switched to another therapy?

The answers are different for those who initially responded to therapy or who are intolerant of therapy than for those who are primary non-responders (Figure 2-1). Patients who were previous responders to their first anti-TNF-α therapy who demonstrate attenuation of that response should be assessed carefully. Is this loss of response or is this due to an infection, stenosis, or irritable bowel? If there is active inflammation present and no infection, the potential explanations for this finding include the development of antibodies and the clearance of drug or loss of response to the mechanism of therapy ("mechanistic escape"). With infliximab, a loss of response can be further assessed with infliximab levels and antibodies to infliximab (ATI). If there is a measurable infliximab level at a trough period of time (immediately before the next scheduled infusion), then this suggests that there may be mechanistic escape and a different class of therapy should be considered. This is when natalizumab[4] or methotrexate may play a role. If the infliximab level is unmeasurable (with or without measurable ATI), pharmacokinetic manipulation with increased doses or decreased intervals of infusions should be attempted to overcome this problem. If the patient has intolerance to infliximab or if pharmacokinetic optimization fails, it is time to consider another drug within the class of anti-TNF therapies.

Some patients losing response or not tolerating infliximab can be successfully switched to adalimumab or certolizumab pegol. The GAIN (Gauging Adalimumab Efficacy in Infliximab Non-Responders) trial evaluated patients who were previously treated with infliximab and became intolerant, or who previously responded and then lost response.[5] Three hundred twenty-five adults with moderate to severe CD were randomized to adalimumab induction therapy versus placebo. Three hundred and one patients completed the trial over a 4-week period of time. The remission rate as defined by a score of less than 150 on the Crohn's Disease Activity Index (CDAI) was 21% versus 7% placebo. Although there is a statistically significant difference, the 21% remission rate is lower than the 32% achieved after induction doses of infliximab in the ACCENT I (A Crohn's Disease Clinical Trial Evaluating Infliximab in a New Long-Term Treatment Regimen) trial,[6] underscoring what has also been seen in rheumatology: that each time a different therapy is tried, the overall response is lower than the first (this is also a word of warning for patients who are stable and still responding to their existing therapy, but wish to switch therapies for "convenience reasons"). It should be noted, however, that the 4-week outcome measured in GAIN improves if these patients are followed for a longer period of time.[7] Other data on patients previously treated with infliximab can be gleaned from the large adalim-

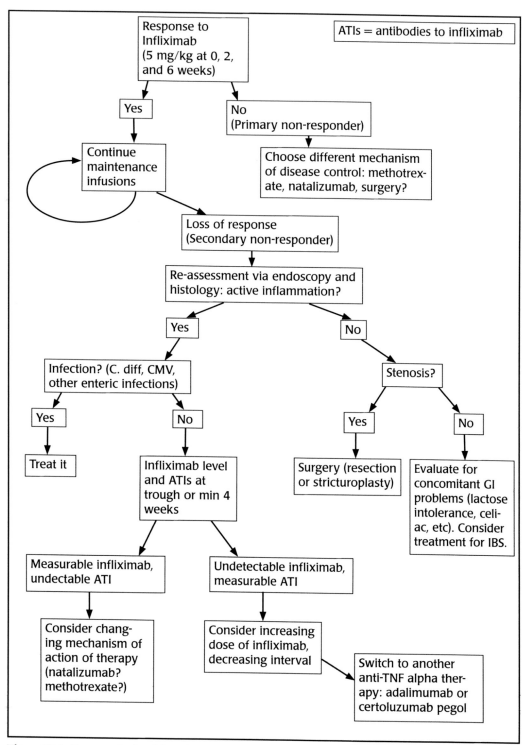

Figure 2-1. Proposed algorithm for assessment of infliximab loss of response. We propose a similar approach if a different anti-TNF-α therapy is used first line, but this has not been fully described yet.

umab and certolizumab pegol clinical trials, CHARM (Crohn's Trial of the Fully Human Antibody Adalimumab for Remission Maintenance) and PRECISE II (The PEGylated Antibody Fragment Evaluation in Crohn's Disease: Safety and Efficacy 2). CHARM is an adalimumab maintenance study in CD patients who responded to adalimumab induction therapy.[8] About 50% of the patients in this trial were previously treated with infliximab. Remission rates ranged from 42% to 48% in the infliximab-naïve patients at 1 year, compared with remission rates of 31% to 34% in the patients who had previously received infliximab. In the PRECISE II trial of maintenance therapy with certolizumab in patients who responded to certolizumab pegol induction, the results were similar.[9] At week 26, the subgroup of patients who were infliximab-naïve had an absolute 100-point response rate (as measured by the CDAI) of 69% as compared to 44% in patients who had previously received infliximab.

A recent case report of 21 patients failing infliximab and treated with open label certolizumab pegol also shows some efficacy.[10] After induction doses at zero and 2 weeks, 43% of patients went into remission at 4 weeks, as measured by the Harvey Bradshaw Index (HBI). The HBI is a validated scale to measure CD activity, and it correlates well with the CDAI in the IBD literature. Among responders, 72% had a previous allergic reaction to infliximab, 50% had a loss of response to infliximab, and 50% were primary non-responders. Similar results without a placebo arm were demonstrated with the certolizumab pegol WELCOME trial (26-Week Open-Label Trial Evaluating the Clinical Benefit and Tolerability of Certolizumab Pegol Induction and Maintenance in Patients Suffering from Crohn's Disease with Prior Loss of Response or Intolerance to Infliximab).[11] Although it is likely, there is not yet data on the reverse direction—switching from adalimumab or certolizumab pegol to infliximab.

There is no published controlled trial that looks at infliximab primary non-responders. At least one-third of patients do not respond initially to infliximab, and many of these have already failed steroids, 6-mercaptopurine (6-MP), azathiorpine, and methotrexate (MTX). Prior to the approval of natalizumab, the only option in this group of patients was surgery. Similar to the evaluation of secondary loss of response above, patients with primary non-response to infliximab should be carefully assessed for strictures, infections, and overlapping irritable bowel syndrome (IBS).

In summary, for patients who initially respond to anti-TNF therapy and then lose response, decrease the interval or increase the dose of infusions or injections, if possible. For infliximab, one can infuse as often as once every 4 weeks with a maximum dose of 10 mg/kg, although the cost-effectiveness of such an approach is unclear. For adalimumab, the maximum published dose is 40 mg each week. No increased dosing regimens for certolizumab pegol have been reported yet. For patients who have lost response to an anti-TNF agent, another anti-TNF agent can be tried. For patients who have lost response to 2 anti-TNF agents, there is no point in trying a third as there is no evidence for efficacy in the medical literature or in clinical practice. For appropriate patients who are allergic or intolerant to infliximab, either adalimumab or certolizumab pegol can be tried. For patients who are primary non-responders to anti-TNF therapy, and for those who have detectable levels of infliximab and demonstrate mechanistic escape, natalizumab is a reasonable option (see Figure 2-1).

References

1. Mackey AC, Green L, Liang LC, Dinnorf P, Avigan M. Hepatosplenic T cell lymphoma associated with infliximab use in young patients treated for inflammatory bowel disease. *J Pediatr Gastroenterol Nutr.* 2007;44(2):265-267.
2. Toruner M, Loftus EV, Harmsen WS, et al. Risk factors for opportunistic infections in patients with inflammatory bowel disease. *Gastroenterology.* 2008;134(4):929-936.
3. Van Assche G, Magdelaine-Beuzelin C, D'Haens G, et al. Withdrawal of azathioprine in patients in remission on infliximab. *Gastroenterology.* 2008;134(7):1861-1868.
4. Sandborn WJ, Colombel JF, Enns R, et al. Natalizumab induction and maintenance therapy for Crohn's disease. *N Engl J Med.* 2005;353(18):1912-1925.
5. Sandborn WJ, Rutgeerts P, Enns R, et al. Adalimumab induction therapy for Crohn's disease previously treated with infliximab: a randomized trial. *Ann Intern Med.* 2007;146(12):829-838.
6. Hanauer S, Feagan BG, Lichtenstein GR, et al. Maintenance infliximab therapy for Crohn's disease: the ACCENT 1 randomized trial. *Lancet.* 2002;359(9317):1541-1549.
7. Panaccione R, Sandborn WJ, D'Haens G, et al. Adalimumab maintains long-term remission in moderately to severely active Crohn's disease after infliximab failure: 1-year follow-up of GAIN trial. *Gastroenterology.* DDW 2008; #920.
8. Colombel JF, Sandborn WJ, Rutgeerts P, et al. Adalimumab for maintenance of clinical response and remission in patients with Crohn's disease: the CHARM trial. *Gastroenterology.* 2007;132(1):52-65.
9. Schreiber S, Khaliq-Kareemi M, Lawrence IC, et al. Maintenance therapy with certolizumab pegol for Crohn's disease. *N Engl J Med.* 2007;357(3):239-250.
10. Danese S, Mocciaro F, Guidi L, et al. Successful induction of clinical response and remission with certolizumab pegol in Crohn's disease patients refractory or intolerant to infliximab: a real-life multicenter experience of compassionate use. *Inflamm Bowel Dis.* 2008;14(8):1168-1170.
11. Vermeire S, Abreu MT, D'Haens G, et al. Efficacy and safety of certolizumab pegol in patients with active Crohn's disease who previously lost response or were intolerant to infliximab: open-label induction preliminary results of the WELCOME study. *Gastroenterology.* DDW 2008; #494.

QUESTION

Is There Ever a Time to Switch 5-Aminosalicyclic Acids in Ulcerative Colitis?

Stephen B. Hanauer, MD, FACG, AGAF

There are several times to switch 5-aminosalicyclic acids (5-ASAs) in ulcerative colitis (UC). Considering that 5-ASAs are the main "foundational" therapies for mild to moderately active disease and for maintaining remissions, it is important to understand the different delivery systems, dosing, and potential side effects.

Despite the variety of oral 5-ASA formulations (azo-bond, pH-dependent, and delayed-delivery), there does not appear to be a substantial difference in efficacy between formulations when administered in equal concentrations of 5-ASA. 5-ASA is a "forgiving molecule" (quote attributed to William Sandborn, MD) with a wide dose range depending upon indication and relatively few side effects at cumulative daily doses up to 8.8 g (4.8 g orally and 4 g rectally). Patients with moderately active disease, those who have been treated with corticosteroids, and those not responding to low doses (less than 2.4 g/day) are more likely to respond to an oral formulation of 4 to 4.8 g. Many patients with left-sided disease will also benefit from a combination of oral and rectal 5-ASA.

The primary consideration when initiating a 5-ASA for UC is the extent of the disease. While in clinical trials of all of the different oral formulations, patients with distal or extensive disease had similar benefits. However, most comparisons between equal doses of oral versus rectal 5-ASA for distal disease suggest that topical therapy is more effective. Hence, one of the most common reasons I would switch between agents would be to change from an oral 5-ASA to a rectal 5-ASA for patients with distal disease that are not responding to an oral agent (or add a rectal agent to the ongoing oral agent).

In other situations, it would be very difficult to demonstrate a differential benefit of changing from one oral formulation to another, aside from patients with unique side effects attributed to the formulation. Most commonly, this would be the case for patients with side effects from the sulfapyridine component of sulfasalazine (sulfa-related intolerance such as rash, allergy, hemolysis, or sperm abnormalities) that are not associated with mesalamine. Other azo-bonded formulations have the propensity to increase colonic secretion in a dose-dependent manner, resulting in increased bowel frequency or liquidity. Substituting a mesalamine formulation may obviate the diarrhea.

In patients who are not responding to an oral 5-ASA, I would consider increasing the dose up to the maximal recommended dose (usually 4 to 4.8 g/day) rather than substituting another agent. Reports of patients improving with one agent after failing another did not take either dose or duration of therapy into consideration. Simply prolonging the duration of therapy is most likely to recruit additional responders. Other case reports of patients improving with one formulation (or tolerating one formulation after intolerance to another) have not been substantiated by prospective studies, aside from comparisons between sulfasalazine and olsalazine, balsalazide, or mesalamine, where sulfasalazine is less well tolerated but numerically, not statistically, superior to the comparator therapy.[1-5]

References

1. Klotz U. Colonic targeting of aminosalicylates for the treatment of ulcerative colitis. *Dig Liver Dis.* 2005;37(6):381-388.
2. Hanauer SB. Review article: aminosalicylates in inflammatory bowel disease. *Aliment Pharmacol Ther.* 2004;20(suppl 4):60-65.
3. Sandborn WJ, Hanauer SB. Systematic review: the pharmacokinetic profiles of oral mesalazine formulations and mesalazine pro-drugs used in the management of ulcerative colitis. *Aliment Pharmacol Ther.* 2003;17(1):29-42.
4. Hanauer SB. Review article: high-dose aminosalicylates to induce and maintain remissions in ulcerative colitis. *Aliment Pharmacol Ther.* 2006;24(suppl 3):37-40.
5. Marteau P, Probert CS, Lindgren S, et al. Combined oral and enema treatment with Pentasa (mesalazine) is superior to oral therapy alone in patients with extensive mild/moderate active ulcerative colitis: a randomized, double blind, placebo controlled study. *Gut.* 2005;54(7):960-965.

WHEN AND HOW DO YOU USE AMINOSALICYLATES IN CROHN'S DISEASE? HOW DO YOU MONITOR RESPONSE TO THERAPY WITH THESE AGENTS?

Stephen B. Hanauer, MD, FACG, AGAF

Despite recent debates in the literature, aminosalicylates have a 30-year history of benefits for mild to moderately active Crohn's disease (CD) in controlled clinical trials. Sulfasalazine was demonstrated to be superior to placebo for patients with colonic involvement in the National Cooperative Crohn's Disease Study (NCCDS), although it was less effective than corticosteroids.[1] Subsequent studies of rectal 5-aminosalicyclic acid (5-ASA) also demonstrated that patients with rectal CD had a clinical response.[2]

Additional uncontrolled and controlled clinical trials have demonstrated several mesalamine formulations to be superior to placebo for the treatment of mild-moderate CD.[3,4] The results for controlled-release mesalamine (Pentasa; Shire, Wayne, PA) have consistently demonstrated that 45% to 55% of patients treated with mesalamine achieved clinical remissions compared to placebo,[5] ciprofloxacin,[6] and budesonide.[7] Furthermore, patients who respond to acute therapy with mesalamine are likely to remain in remission with continued maintenance therapy.[8]

The problems with interpreting studies regarding mesalamine in CD include different patient populations, baseline medications, and disease severity. In particular, patients enrolled into maintenance studies have been quite heterogeneous, and many of the trials had high placebo responses.[9-11] An important issue related to mesalamine as a maintenance therapy depends upon what agent induced remission. It does appear that after corticosteroid induction, mesalamine is no more effective than placebo (about 20%) at maintaining remissions.[12]

The current monitoring of patients is clinical, taking into account patients' symptoms, signs, laboratory data (hemoglobin, albumin), extraintestinal complications, and quality of life. I use the American College of Gastroenterology (ACG) clinical criteria to assess the overall status.[13] Mucosal healing, while appealing, is not a current standard to assess medical therapy for CD.

Thus, I continue to advocate aminosalicylates for mildly active CD for patients with ileal and/or colonic disease. I then monitor the clinical response. If patients improve and have a resolution of their symptoms and signs, I continue therapy as long as they are responding. I usually use another agent such as budesonide for patients with more moderate ileal and/or ascending colon disease, or I use a short course of systemic corticosteroids. If patients lose response to mesalamine, or if they required corticosteroids to gain control, I will use an alternative agent.

References

1. Summers RW, Switz DM, Sessions JT Jr, et al. National Cooperative Crohn's Disease Study: results of drug treatment. *Gastroenterology*. 1979;77(4, pt 2):847-869.
2. Klotz U, Maier K, Fischer C, Heinkel K. Therapeutic efficacy of sulfasalazine and its metabolites in patients with ulcerative colitis and Crohn's disease. *N Engl J Med*. 1980;303(26):1499-1502.
3. Singleton JW, Hanauer SB, Gitnick GL, et al. Mesalamine capsules for the treatment of active Crohn's disease: results of a 16-week trial. Pentasa Crohn's Disease Study Group. *Gastroenterology*. 1993;104(5):1293-1301.
4. Tremaine WJ, Schroeder KW, Harrison JM, Zinsmeister AR. A randomized, double-blind, placebo-controlled trial of the oral mesalamine (5-ASA) preparation, Asacol, in the treatment of symptomatic Crohn's colitis and ileocolitis. *J Clin Gastroenterol*. 1994;19(4):278-282.
5. Hanauer SB, Stromberg U. Oral Pentasa in the treatment of active Crohn's disease: a meta-analysis of double-blind, placebo-controlled trials. *Clin Gastroenterol Hepatol*. 2004;2(5):379-388.
6. Colombel JF, Lemann M, Cassagnou M, et al. A controlled trial comparing ciprofloxacin with mesalazine for the treatment of active Crohn's disease. Groupe d'Etudes Therapeutiques des Affections Inflammatoires Digestives (GETAID). *Am J Gastroenterol*. 1999;94(3):674-678.
7. Thomsen OO, Cortot A, Jewell D, et al. A comparison of budesonide and mesalamine for active Crohn's disease. International Budesonide-Mesalamine Study Group. *N Engl J Med*. 1998;339(6):370-374.
8. Hanauer SB, Krawitt EL, Robinson M, Rick GG, Safdi MA. Long-term management of Crohn's disease with mesalamine capsules (Pentasa). Pentasa Crohn's Disease Compassionate Use Study Group. *Am J Gastroenterol*. 1993;88(9):1343-1351.
9. Su C, Lichtenstein GR, Krok K, Brensinger CM, Lewis JD. A meta-analysis of the placebo rates of remission and response in clinical trials of active Crohn's disease. *Gastroenterology*. 2004;126(5):1257-1269.
10. Steinhart AH, Forbes A, Mills EC, Rodgers-Gray BS, Travis SP. Systematic review: the potential influence of mesalazine formulation on maintenance of remission in Crohn's disease. *Aliment Pharmacol Ther*. 2007;25(12):1389-1399.
11. van Bodegraven AA, Mulder CJ. Indications for 5-aminosalicylate in inflammatory bowel disease: is the body of evidence complete? *World J Gastroenterol*. 2006;12(38):6115-6123.
12. Gendre JP, Mary JY, Florent C, et al. Oral mesalamine (Pentasa) as maintenance treatment in Crohn's disease: a multicenter placebo-controlled study. The Groupe d'Etudes Therapeutiques des Affections Inflammatoires Digestives (GETAID). *Gastroenterology*. 1993;104(2):435-439.
13. Hanauer SB, Sandborn W. Management of Crohn's disease in adults. *Am J Gastroenterol*. 2001;96(3):635-643.

QUESTION

WHAT IS THE ROLE OF CONCOMITANT IMMUNOMODULATORS WITH BIOLOGIC USE IN INFLAMMATORY BOWEL DISEASE?

Mark Lazarev, MD and Miguel Regueiro, MD

Immunomodulators such as azathioprine and 6-mercaptopurine (6-MP) have traditionally been used as maintenance therapy for patients with moderate to severe Crohn's disease (CD) and ulcerative colitis (UC). However, a certain proportion of patients are intolerant to or fail to respond to immunomodulators and require a biologic agent. Anti-tumor necrosis factor (TNF) agents (infliximab, adalimumab, certolizumab) are biologic agents currently available for inflammatory bowel disease (IBD) and are effective at inducing and maintaining remission in CD and UC (infliximab). Whether anti-TNF agents should be used as monotherapy or in combination with immunomodulators is the question. Really, there are 3 questions that have emerged on this topic:

1. Do concomitant immunomodulators impact on immunogenicity (ie, antibody formation against the biologic)?

2. Is the concomitant use of immunomodulators with a biologic agent safe?

3. Are concomitant immunomodulators necessary to improve the efficacy of biologics?

The answer to the first question is: *Yes, concomitant immunomodulator use does decrease immunogenicity of biologic therapy.* It is a fact that all anti-TNF agents are foreign proteins and cause a certain percentage of people to produce antibodies against the biologic agent, hence they are immunogenic. We know that the concomitant use of immunomodulators decreases immunogenicity of biologic agents. This was shown in a study by Baert and a separate study by Vermeire. In the study by Baert et al, 125 patients with CD were given an induction course of infliximab at zero, 2, and 6 weeks, followed by episodic infusions for clinical relapse.[1] A significantly higher percentage (75%) of patients on episodic infliximab monotherapy developed antibodies to infliximab (ATIs) compared with those on concomitant immunomodulators (43%). Vermeire et al found similar rates of ATI

15

formation in patients receiving episodic infliximab monotherapy compared to those on concomitant immunomodulators (either methotrexate [MTX] or azathioprine).[2] These studies evaluated immunogenicity in patients receiving episodic infliximab. However, it has become the practice of most gastroenterologists to use regularly scheduled (every 8 weeks) maintenance infusions. So, what is the immunogenicity in patients receiving regularly scheduled maintenance infusions with or without immunomodulators? In the ACCENT I (A Crohn's Disease Clinical Trial Evaluating Infliximab in a New Long-Term Treatment Regimen) study, CD patients received maintenance infliximab infusions every 8 weeks after the initial 3 induction doses.[3] The immunogenicity rate was much lower than previously reported in the episodic studies and did not significantly change between those on concomitant immunomodulators and those on infliximab monotherapy (10.9% ATI formation in patients on infliximab monotherapy versus 6.7% in those on concomitant immunomodulators).[4] In summary, concomitant immunomodulator use decreases immunogenicity to infliximab in patients receiving episodic treatment. Patients receiving maintenance infusions every 8-weeks, regardless of concomitant immunomodulators, had lower rates of ATI formation.

The answer to the second question is: *Usually—immunomodulators in combination with a biologic agent are usually safe.* Data from the TREAT (Crohn's Therapy Resource, Evaluation, and Assessment Tool) registry, a post-marketing data set that tracks adverse events related to infliximab, has provided additional safety information in IBD patients.[5] The risk of opportunistic infection, cancer, and lymphoma remains low in infliximab-treated patients. Immunomodulators have also rarely been linked to infection and malignancy. One meta-analysis showed an increased relative risk (RR) of lymphoma (RR = 4.18, 95% Confidence Interval [CI] 2.07 – 7.51).[6] To date, there have been 13 patients with CD who developed hepatosplenic T-cell lymphoma (HSTCL).[7] This usually fatal disease has been found in adolescents and young adults. All of the patients were on infliximab and azathioprine/6-MP. There have been no cases reported in patients on infliximab alone or in those on MTX in combination with infliximab. However, there have been reported cases of HSTCL in patients on azathioprine/6-MP without infliximab. Given that HSTCL has only occurred in patients treated with azathioprine/6-MP, infliximab monotherapy may be reasonable on the basis of safety data alone.

The answer to the third question is: *In some cases immunomodulators may improve the efficacy of biologics.* In a meta-analysis by Lichtenstein et al, the 54-week response and remission rates in the infliximab CD maintenance study (ACCENT I) and the Active Ulcerative Colitis Trial (ACT I + II) studies were not statistically different between patients with and without concomitant immunomodulators.[8] To determine whether infliximab-treated patients can stop their concomitant immunomodulators and maintain remission, van Assche et al randomized 80 CD patients who were in remission on infliximab and an immunomodulator for at least 6 months to 2 arms: one that would continue their concomitant immunomodulator, and the other that would stop their immunomodulator.[9] At the end of 2 years, the same proportion of patients were in clinical and endoscopic remission, suggesting that infliximab monotherapy was as effective as the combination with an immunomodulator (Figure 5-1). Similarly, a study by Colombel et al did not show a difference in 1 year remission rates for patients treated with adalimumab monotherapy compared with those on concomitant immunomodulators.[10]

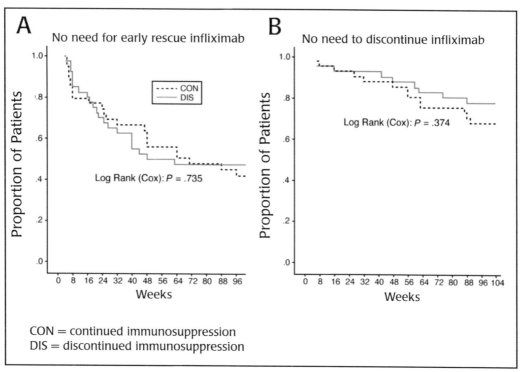

Figure 5-1. Crohn's disease: withdrawal of immunosuppression in patients treated with scheduled maintenance infliximab. Reprinted from *Gastroenterology*, 134(7), van Assche G, Magdelaine–Beuzelin C, D'Haens G, et al. Withdrawal of immunosuppression in Crohn's disease treated with scheduled infliximab maintenance: a randomized trial, p. 8, Copyright (2008), with permission from Elsevier.

Most recently, Sandborn et al presented data at the American College of Gastroenterology (ACG) from the 2008 SONIC (Study of Immunomodulator-Naive Patients in Crohn's Disease) trial.[11] This is the first prospective trial of its kind to compare monotherapy with combination therapy. The study population included 508 patients with moderate to severe steroid-dependent CD who had no prior exposure to immunomodulators or biologic agents. Patients were randomized to receive one of the following:

- azathioprine 2.5 mg/kg + placebo infusions
- infliximab 5 mg/kg + placebo capsules
- infliximab 5 mg/kg + azathioprine 2.5 mg/kg.

The primary endpoint was corticosteroid-free remission at week 26. This endpoint was achieved in 30.6% of patients who received azathioprine alone, 44.4% who received infliximab alone, and 56.8% of those who received combination therapy (Figure 5-2). Results were statistically significant between all 3 arms. Subgroup analysis revealed particularly robust findings in patients with a C-reactive protein (CRP) > 0.8 mg/dL or lesions on baseline endoscopy.

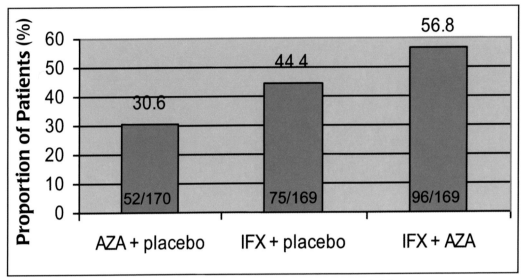

Figure 5-2. SONIC trial. Corticosteroid-free clinical remission at week 26.

In our practice, the role of concomitant immunomodulators with biologics is as follows:

- For CD patients in remission for more than 6 months on infliximab and concomitant immunomodulators, we lower the immunomodulator dose. If the patient continues to do well, we stop the immunomodulator and continue infliximab monotherapy.

- For CD patients who are steroid-dependent and naïve to immunomodulators or biologic agents, it may now be reasonable to institute concomitant therapy.

- For CD patients treated with adalimumab, we do not use concomitant immunomodulators.

- For UC patients on an immunomodulator at the time infliximab is started, we continue the immunomodulator until remission is achieved, and then stop the immunomodulator and continue infliximab monotherapy.

- For UC patients not on an immunomodulator at the time infliximab is started, we do not use concomitant immunomodulators.

Therefore, based on the safety data and the fact that combining immunologic agents probably leads to an increased risk of complications, biologic therapy without concomitant immunomodulators is reasonable in most cases. Long-term efficacy data are needed to determine whether stopping immunomodulators negatively impacts the biologic response and remission rates. It is our practice to restart the immunomodulator in patients who reactivate their disease in the setting of biologic monotherapy.

References

1. Baert F, Noman M, Vermeire S, et al. Influence of immunogenicity on the long-term efficacy of infliximab in Crohn's disease. *N Engl J Med.* 2003;348(7):601-608.
2. Vermeire S, Noman M, Van Assche G, Baert F, D'Haens G, Rutgeerts P. Effectiveness of concomitant immunosuppressive therapy in suppressing the formation of antibodies to infliximab in Crohn's disease. *Gut.* 2007;56(9):1226-1231.
3. Hanauer SB, Feagan BG, Lichtenstein GR, et al. Maintenance infliximab for Crohn's disease: the ACCENT I randomized trial. *Lancet.* 2002;359(9317):1541-1549.
4. Hanauer SB, Wagner CL, Bala M, et al. Incidence and importance of antibody responses to infliximab after maintenance or episodic treatment in Crohn's disease. *Clin Gastroenterol Hepatol.* 2004;2(7):542-553.
5. Lichtenstein GR, Feagan BG, Cohen RD, et al. Serious infections and mortality in association with therapies for Crohn's disease: TREAT registry. *Clin Gastroenterol Hepatol.* 2006;4(5):621-630.
6. Kandiel A, Fraser AG, Korelitz BI, Brensinger C, Lewis JD. Increased risk of lymphoma among inflammatory bowel disease patients treated with azathioprine and 6-mercaptopurine. *Gut.* 2005;54(8):1121-1125.
7. Mackey AC, Green L, Liang LC, Dinndorf P, Avigan M. Hepatosplenic T cell lymphoma associated with infliximab use in young patients treated for inflammatory bowel disease. *J Pediatr Gastroenterol Nutr.* 2007;44(2):265-267.
8. Lichtenstein GR, Diamond RH, Wagner C, et al. Infliximab administered as 3-dose induction followed by scheduled maintenance therapy in IBD: comparable clinical outcomes with or without concomitant immunomodulators. *Gastroenterology.* 2007;132(suppl 2):A-146.
9. Van Assche G, Magdelaine-Beuzelin C, D'Haens G, et al. Withdrawal of immunosuppression in Crohn's disease treated with scheduled infliximab maintenance: a randomized trial. *Gastroenterology.* 2008;134:1861-1868.
10. Colombel JF, Sandborn WJ, Rutgeerts P, et al. Adalimumab for maintenance of clinical response and remission in patients with Crohn's disease: the CHARM trial. *Gastroenterology.* 2007;132(1):52-65.
11. Sandborn W, Rutgeerts P, Reinisch W, et al. SONIC: A randomized, double-blind, controlled trial comparing infliximab and infliximab plus azathioprine to azathioprine in patients with Crohn's disease naïve to immunomodulators and biologic therapy. *Am J Gastroenterology.* 2008;103(suppl 1):S436.

QUESTION

WHAT NEW DRUGS HAVE RECENTLY BEEN RELEASED TO TREAT INFLAMMATORY BOWEL DISEASE? WHAT NEW DRUGS CAN WE ANTICIPATE BEING RELEASED IN THE NEXT 5 YEARS? HOW WILL THEY CHANGE OUR TREATMENT ALGORITHMS?

Remo Panaccione, MD, FRCPC

Several agents have recently joined our therapeutic armamentarium in the treatment of inflammatory bowel disease (IBD). Two new agents have joined the anti-tumor necrosis factor (TNF) class, which has proven to be successful, while others are directed against new targets.

ANTI–TUMOR NECROSIS FACTOR-ALPHA THERAPY

Infliximab ushered in the era of anti-TNF therapy in IBD when it was approved for the treatment of moderately to severely active luminal Crohn's disease (CD) by the Food and Drug Administration (FDA) in 1998. Since then, infliximab has been approved for the treatment of fistulas in CD, pediatric CD, and for the treatment of ulcerative colitis (UC). Recently, the fully human monoclonal antibody adalimumab (Humira; Abbott Laboratories, Abbott Park, IL) and the pegylated humanized monoclonal antibody certolizumab pegol (Cimzia; UCB Inc, Brussels, Belgium) also have been approved for the treatment of moderately to severely active luminal CD.

21

Adalimumab was approved for CD in February 2007, and certolizumab pegol was approved in April 2008. Adalimumab is a fully human IgG1 antibody to TNF-alpha (α), and certolizumab pegol is made up of the Fab fragment of a humanized monoclonal antibody to TNF-α linked with 2 molecules of polyethylene glycol. Since it lacks the FC portion of the antibody, certolizumab pegol only exerts its activity through binding to soluble TNF-α, and cannot bind to cell surface receptors. In PRECISE II (Pegylated Antibody Fragment Evaluation in Crohn's Disease: Safety and Efficacy), 668 patients with moderately to severely active CD received open label certolizumab pegol 400 mg at weeks zero, 2, and 4.[1] Responders (decrease in Crohn's disease Activity Index [CDAI] of 100 points) were then randomized to either continue to receive certolizumab pegol 400 mg SC (subcutaneous injection) every 4 weeks or placebo every 4 weeks. The primary endpoint was the proportion of patients able to maintain response through week 26. Patients were stratified according to baseline CRP, immunosuppressant use, and cortico-steroid use. Sixty-four percent of patients responded to the initial induction dosing. These patients were then randomized 1:1 to placebo or certolizumab pegol. At week 26, 62.8% of the certolizumab pegol-treated patients maintained response, compared to 36.2% of patients randomized to placebo ($p < 0.001$). The proportion of patients who were able to remain in remission was also significantly higher in those receiving certolizumab pegol (47.9% versus 28.6%; $p < 0.001$). There were no differences in this study amongst patients with elevated CRP, those taking concomitant immunosuppressives, or those previously exposed to anti-TNF therapy.

In a second phase III trial (the PRECISE 1 study), a placebo-controlled phase III trial was designed to evaluate the efficacy and tolerability of SC-administered certolizumab pegol 400 mg for the induction and maintenance of clinical response and remission in patients with moderately to severely active CD.[2] A substantial proportion of patients in the PRECISE 1 trial had received prior treatment with infliximab (28%). In this study, 659 patients were initially randomized to receive placebo ($n = 328$) or certolizumab pegol ($n = 331$) beginning at week zero, and continued receiving treatment for 26 weeks, regardless of their response to treatment at week 6. As a result, all patients in the trial were evaluated for efficacy and safety throughout the 26-week study. Results from the PRECISE 1 study demonstrated that clinical response rates were significantly higher ($p < 0.05$) throughout the 26-week treatment period in patients in the intent-to-treat population who received treatment with certolizumab pegol 400 mg when compared with the rates in patients who were randomized to the placebo arm. A significant difference in response rates was observed as early as week 4 (29% with certolizumab pegol versus 22% with placebo; $p < 0.05$) and the difference in response rates between the 2 treatment arms was essentially the same at week 26 (35% versus 27%, respectively; $p < 0.05$). The percentage of patients who achieved a clinical response at both week 6 and week 26 were slightly lower in each treatment arm than the percentages observed at individual time points (23% versus 16%, respectively), although the difference in rates between the 2 treatment arms was still statistically significant ($p \leq 0.05$). The difference in clinical remission rates between the 2 treatment arms in the intent-to-treat population was significant only at week 4 (20% with certolizumab pegol versus 11% with placebo; $p \leq 0.01$).

Adalimumab and certolizumab pegol are currently being studied for the treatment of UC. Finally, golimumab, another fully human monoclonal antibody against TNF-α that can be administered as either a SC injection or intravenous (IV) infusion is being investigated for the treatment of both CD and UC.

INHIBITORS OF LEUKOCYTE ADHESION

Integrins are expressed on the surface of leukocytes and serve as mediators of leukocyte adhesion to vascular endothelium. Alpha4 (α4) integrins along with its beta1 (ß1) or ß7 subunit interact with endothelial ligands, termed *adhesion molecules*. Interaction between α4ß7 and mucosal addressin cellular adhesion molecule (MAdCAM-1) is important in lymphocyte trafficking to gut mucosa. Natalizumab (Tysabri; Biogen Idec, Inc, Cambridge, MA) is a recombinant humanized immunoglobulin G4 (IgG4) antibody against α4 integrin that has been shown to be effective in the induction and maintenance of patients with CD. It was approved in February 2008 for the treatment of patients with CD refractory or intolerant to anti-TNF-α therapy.

In the ENACT-1 (Evaluation of Natalizumab in Active Crohn's disease Therapy 1) trial, 905 patients were randomized to 300 mg or placebo at weeks zero, 4, and 8.[3] The primary outcome was clinical response (decrease in CDAI of > 70 points) at week 10. Both natalizumab 300 mg and placebo had similar rates of response and remission at 12 weeks. Response was 56% and 49%, and 37% and 30% for remission in treatment and control group at week 10, respectively. However, subgroup analysis found significant differences in both response and remission rates in patients with an elevated C-reactive protein (CRP) at baseline and/or on concomitant immunomodulators. Among patients with a CRP > 2.87 mg/L, the clinical response was 58% in the natalizumab group and 45% in the placebo group (p = .007) with clinical remission in 40% and 28%, respectively (p = .014). Given these findings, the ENCORE (Efficacy of Natalizumab in Crohn's Disease Response and Remission) trial studied only patients with an elevated CRP and moderately to severely active CD.[4] The primary endpoint required a sustained response at week 8 through week 12 of > 70 decrease in CDAI after 3 infusions every 4 hours with either natalizumab at 300 mg or placebo. In this study, patients on natalizumab had a significantly higher rate of sustained response (48%) compared to placebo (32%) (p < .001). Rates of sustained remission were also higher in the natalizumab group (26%) compared to the placebo group (16%) (p = 0.002).

Furthermore, natalizumab has been shown to have clinical efficacy in the maintenance of remission. In the ENACT-2 study, 354 patients who had a response to natalizumab in ENACT-1 were enrolled into maintenance therapy with an infusion of natalizumab or placebo every 4 weeks through week 56.[3] The primary outcome was a sustained response through week 36 with a secondary outcome of disease remission. Sixty-one percent of the patients in the natalizumab arm achieved sustained response versus 28% in the placebo group, which was statistically significant (p < .001). Similarly, natalizumab-treated patients were more likely to be in remission through week 36 (44% versus 26%, p = .003). Also, there was a steroid-sparing effect with 45% of the patients on natalizumab who were in remission and corticosteroid-free, compared to 22% of the patients in the placebo group. However, one patient died from progressive multifocal leukoencephalopathy (PML) associated with the JC polyoma virus in the open label extension part of the trial. An additional 2 cases of PML were diagnosed in patients on natalizumab for multiple sclerosis (MS). This resulted in the withdrawal of natalizumab from the market for MS and from further development in other disease areas. On June 5, 2006, the US Food and Drug Administration (FDA) approved a Supplemental Biologics License Application (sBLA) for the reintroduction of natalizumab as monotherapy treatment for relapsing forms of

MS. The reintroduction is under the auspices of the TOUCH (Tysabri Outreach: Unified Commitment to Health) pharmacovigilence program due to the previous cases of PML.

In December 2006, the sponsor filed a supplemental license application with the FDA for the treatment of CD with natalizumab. On July 31, 2007, the Gastrointestinal Drugs and Drug Safety and Risk Management Advisory Committees of the Food and Drug Administration (FDA) recommended the approval of natalizumab for the treatment of moderately to severely active CD patients who have failed or cannot tolerate available therapies, including anti-TNF-α therapy. The FDA reapproved natalizumab in February 2008 under the TOUCH prescribing program. This program details strict criteria that doctors and patients must adhere to, including not using concomitant immunomodulators, tapering steroids by 6 months of treatment, signing consent forms, and a monthly check by the infusion nurses for signs and symptoms of PML. As of November 2008, over 48,000 patients have been infused with natalizumab for both Crohn's disease and MS, and there have been a total of 6 reported cases of PML. The 3 post-marketing cases have occurred in patients with MS who were receiving monotherapy. All were treated with plamapharesis and anti-viral therapy. Although there is considerable morbidity, no further patients have died.

OTHER THERAPIES IN DEVELOPMENT

Since TNF-α, other cytokines have been implicated in the IBD-related inflammatory process. Although likely to be overly simplistic, the classic paradigm for cytokine involvement in the pathogenesis of CD includes the hypothesis that excess cytokine activity mediated by type 1 helper T (Th1) cells and Interleukin-12 (IL-12), derived from intestinal antigen presenting cells, initiates Th-1-mediated inflammation. Mannon et al, in a double-blind randomized controlled trial, evaluated the safety and efficacy of a human monoclonal antibody against IL-12.[5] Seventy-nine patients with moderately active CD were randomly assigned to receive 7 weekly injections of anti–IL-12 (1 or 3 mg/kg of body weight) or placebo, and were then followed for 18 weeks. With the exception of local injection site reactions, there were no significant differences in the rate of adverse events between intervention and placebo groups. The results of the trial suggest that clinical response and remission could be rapid in onset and durable. Patients receiving the uninterrupted weekly injections of anti-IL-12 3 mg/kg achieved higher response rates than placebo (75% versus 25%, $p = 0.03$). IL-23 is a cytokine composed of p19 and p20 protein subunits, which is also up-regulated in CD mucosa. Therefore, IL-23 biological activity could be inhibited by neutralizing IL-12 p40 antibodies, raising the question of whether the observed benefit of anti-IL-12 therapy is due to its neutralizing effect on IL-12 or IL-23. The recent discovery of IL-23 as an IBD gene from a genome-wide association study strengthens the case against IL-23 as an important signalling pathway and therapeutic target in IBD. CNTO 1275 is a fully human monoclonal antibody targeting the common p40 subunit of IL-12 and IL-23. In a 14-week phase II study,[6] the safety and efficacy of either a single IV infusion or 4 SC injections of CNTO 1275 were evaluated in patients with moderate to severe CD, including non-responders to infliximab. Clinical response was defined as a reduction from baseline in the CDAI of $\geq 25\%$ and ≥ 70 points. At week 8, 49.0% of patients receiving CNTO 1275 were in clinical response versus 39.6% who received placebo ($p = .34$; primary end point). At week 4 and at week 6, a total of 52.9% of patients receiving CNTO 1275 were in clinical response versus 30.2% receiving placebo ($p = .02$). Forty-nine percent of patients receiving CNTO 1275 were in response at week 8 using $\geq$ 100-point CDAI reduction from baseline versus 30.2% receiving placebo ($p = .05$). For patients who had previous infliximab exposure, 59.1% who received CNTO 1275 were in clinical response at week 8, compared with 25.9% who received placebo ($p = .02$). The study authors concluded that short-term treatment with this novel monoclonal antibody was generally well tolerated and had a beneficial effect in patients with moderate to severe CD. There is a phase III trial now in progress.

Changing Paradigms

It is likely that the introduction of new therapies will change treatment paradigms in IBD. Within the anti-TNF-α class, there will be increasing use of the SC preparations, likely as a result of increased convenience to patients. There will be increased interest in which patients will benefit from earlier introduction of these agents, with the potential for improved outcomes. The positioning of newer agents, either as monotherapy or in combination with others, remains to be determined.

References

1. Sandborn WJ, Feagan BG, Stoinov S, et al. Certolizumab pegol for the treatment of Crohn's disease. *N Engl J Med.* 2007;357(3):228-238.
2. Schreiber S, Khaliq-Kareemi M, Lawrance IC, et al. Maintenance therapy with certolizumab pegol for Crohn's disease. *N Engl J Med.* 2007;357(3):239-250.
3. Sandborn WJ, Colombel JF, Enns R, et al. Natalizumab induction and maintenance therapy for Crohn's disease. *N Engl J Med.* 2005;353(18):1912-1925.
4. Targan SR, Feagan BG, Fedorak RN, et al. Natalizumab for the treatment of active Crohn's disease: results of the ENCORE trial. *Gastroenterology.* 2007;132(5):1672-1683.
5. Mannon PJ, Fuss IJ, Mayer L, et al. Anti-interleukin-12 antibody for active Crohn's disease. *N Engl J Med.* 2004;351(20):2069-2079.
6. Sandborn WJ, Feagan BG, Fedorak RN, et al. A randomized trial of Ustekinumab, a human interleukin-12/23 monoclonal antibody, in patients with moderate-to-severe Crohn's disease. *Gastroenterology.* 2008;135(4):1130-1141.

risk attributable to infliximab.[2] In contrast, a population-based Swedish study estimated a 2% risk of lymphoma, and a single-center experience from the Mayo Clinic reported a 1% risk of death attributable to infliximab.[3,4] A systematic review of the literature included over 1700 patients treated with infliximab from 6 studies, and developed a summary estimate describing an annual risk of lymphoma of 0.2% (20/10,000), and a 0.4% (4/10,000) risk of dying from sepsis related to infliximab (Table 7-1).[5] A recent meta-analysis of the risk of non-Hodgkin's lymphoma with anti-TNF agents predicts a lower rate at 0.055% (5.5/10,000), which is approximately 3 times higher than expected in the general population, and 1.5 times higher than a comparator group of patients taking 6-mercaptopurine (6-MP) or azathioprine.

Hepatosplenic T-cell lymphoma (HSTCL) is a recently described, nearly universally fatal lymphoma in patients with Crohn's disease (CD) taking immunomodulators and anti-TNF agents. At least 3 cases involved immunomodulators alone, and 12 cases received combination therapy. Patients tended to be young (mean age 21), and almost all have been male. Due to the uncertainty of how many patients in this age range have received immunomodulators and anti-TNF agents, it is not possible to estimate the rate of occurrence. It appears to be a very rare yet real problem that requires further attention. We should inform patients about this, reinforce how unusual it is, and make individual patient-based decisions to determine if biologic therapy is necessary and if concomitant immunomodulators are required.

The uncertainty undermining the data on the risk of biologics is not limited to the wide range of estimates in the literature. Risk factors for serious adverse events among persons receiving infliximab are unknown. The contributions from other medications, co-morbid disease, and duration of treatment have yet to be defined. Furthermore, current estimates of risk are primarily annual risks. Lifetime risks are unknown, and it is not clear if the risks are cumulative. Acknowledging these uncertainties is important to convey the data appropriately.

Other rare but serious potential events associated with infliximab, including congestive heart failure, hepatic failure, solid tumors, drug-induced lupus, pancytopenia, and tuberculosis, also deserve specific mention when introducing the concept of biologic therapy. With the exception of tuberculosis (see Table 7-1), the frequency of these conditions is unknown and likely too low to adequately quantitate. When presenting to patients, it is reasonable simply to explain that these events are very rare and probably occur less often than sepsis.

BALANCING RISKS AND BENEFITS

For physicians, knowing whether the benefits indeed outweigh risks is often more complex than it might seem. With this in mind, a decision analytic model was developed to help understand the trade-off between risks and benefits of infliximab for CD.[5] The simulated clinical trial of 200,000 hypothetical patients compared infliximab to standard therapy, including surgery, immunomodulators, and steroids. Despite an increase in lymphoma and death from sepsis, the overall quality of life was higher in the infliximab arm due to the large proportion of subjects who experienced clinical improvement (based on a 60% response rate and 20% end-of-year remission rate as was seen in the ACCENT 1 [A Crohn's Disease Clinical Trial Evaluating Infliximab in a New Long-Term Treatment Regimen] trial).[6]

Table 7-1
Serious Side Effects of Anti-TNF Agents in Crohn's Disease

Event	Estimated Frequency (annual)
NHL (baseline)	0.02% (2/10,000)¶
NHL (on IM)	0.04% (4/10,000)*
NHL (on anti-TNF)	0.06% (6/10,000)^
HSTCL	unknown
Death from sepsis	0.4% (4/1000)#
Tuberculosis	0.05% (5/10,000)~

Adapted from Siegel CA. Comprehensive approach to patient risk. Risk versus benefit of biologics and immune suppressants. In: Targan S, Shanahan F, Karp L, eds. *Inflammatory Bowel Disease: Translating Basic Science into Clinical Practice.* In press, 2009.

¶ Frequency of NHL in Surveillance Epidemiology End Results registry, all ages
* Frequency of NHL in Crohn's patients on immunomodulators
   from Kandiel et al 2005 meta-analysis
^ Frequency of NHL in Crohn's patients on anti-TNF agents
   from Siegel meta-analysis (personal communication)
Estimate from Siegel et al 2005 meta-analysis
~ Data on file, Centocor, Inc.

TNF = tumor necrosis factor
NHL = non-Hodgkin's lymphoma
IM = immunomodulator (azathioprine/6-mercaptopurine)
HSTCL = hepatosplenic T-cell lymphoma

The inherent uniqueness of each patient makes generic statements like "benefits outweigh risks" inappropriate, as each patient has a different level of symptoms and a personal threshold of how much risk he or she is willing to take. Factors that affect patients' risk thresholds have been described in a recent study. As the severity of disease increases and the promised benefit of treatment increases, not surprisingly, patients will take higher risks than have been reported in the literature for lymphoma, death from infections, and progressive multifocal leukoencephalopathy.[7]

Given that patients will adjust their risk thresholds depending on the clinical situation, it is vital that their perceptions of the risks and benefits are accurate. A study evaluating patients' understanding of biologic therapy showed that they tended to underestimate the risks and overestimate the benefits of infliximab. More concerning, when a hypothetical "new drug" with risks of lymphoma and death approximating infliximab was described to patients, over two-thirds said they would refuse the medicine. One-third of these patients had taken or were currently taking infliximab.[8] The onus of communicating the risks and benefits and ensuring that patients understand them is on the clinician, and new approaches may be needed to ensure this is done more effectively.

COMMUNICATING RISKS TO PATIENTS

Effectively communicating risk is challenging. Reviewing the risks encountered in daily life and the inherent risks of IBD may help patients gain perspective. For example, the lifetime risk of developing lymphoma in the general population is 1 in 50.[9] Approximately 1 in 5 patients with CD will require surgery within the first year of diagnosis, and 4 in 5 will require surgery over 20 years of disease. Because these risks are part of life and part of the diagnosis of IBD, they are often more accepted. Knowingly assuming risks of medications is perceived as an optional risk, and even a small added risk may prove unappealing to patients.

Framing is the unintentional (or perhaps intentional) presentation of data in such a way to influence a decision. Not surprisingly, patients will change their preferences when risks are framed in absolute (eg, "a 2% risk reduction" to describe a decrease of risk from 4% to 2%) versus relative risk (RR) reductions (eg, "a 50% decreased risk"). Care should be taken to avoid framing and to present data as accurately as possible. Presenting risks as an absolute number over a common denominator is probably the most effective, and giving a range when there is uncertainty is appropriate. For example, the annual risk of lymphoma in the general population is about 2/10,000 persons, and the risk of lymphoma while on infliximab is between 5/10,000 and 20/10,000. Practical tips for presenting risk are outlined in Table 7-2.

CONCLUSION

As more biologics are approved for the treatment of IBD, and as they are used earlier in the disease course, understanding the risks becomes more important. Involving our patients in choosing appropriate therapies and ensuring that the risks are communicated clearly will become even more critical as treatment algorithms evolve. To best deliver this information to our patients, we need to carefully review the available evidence, endeavor to put it into perspective for our patients, focus on the most serious risks of biologics, avoid framing, and invite patients to be involved in these preference-based decisions.

Table 7-2

Practical Considerations in Presenting Risk to Patients

1. Acknowledge uncertainty of the data.
2. Present data as absolute risk (X out of 100; 1000; 10,000).
3. Attempt to keep denominators consistent.
4. Avoid framing.
5. Present risk in the context of other life (and disease-related) risks.
6. Don't overwhelm patients with too much data. Focus on the most important information.

References

1. Remicade (infliximab) for IV injection (prescribing information). 2008. Available at: http://www.centocor. com/centocor/assets/remicade.pdf. Accessed January 18, 2009.
2. Lichtenstein GR, Feagan BG, Cohen RD, et al. Serious infections and mortality in association with therapies for Crohn's disease: TREAT registry. *Clin Gastroenterol Hepatol.* 2006;4(5):621-630.
3. Ljung T, Karlen P, Schmidt D, et al. Infliximab in inflammatory bowel disease: clinical outcome in a population based cohort from Stockholm County. *Gut.* 2004;53(6):849-853.
4. Colombel JF, Loftus EV Jr, Tremaine WJ, et al. The safety profile of infliximab in patients with Crohn's disease: the Mayo clinic experience in 500 patients. *Gastroenterology.* 2004;126(1):19-31.
5. Siegel CA, Hur C, Korzenik JR, Gazelle GS, Sands BE. Risks and benefits of infliximab for the treatment of Crohn's disease. *Clin Gastroenterol Hepatol.* 2006;4(8):1017-1024.
6. Hanauer SB, Feagan BG, Lichtenstein GR, et al. Maintenance infliximab for Crohn's disease: the ACCENT I randomized trial. *Lancet.* 2002;359(9317):1541-1549.
7. Johnson F, Ozdemir S, Mansfield C, et al. Crohn's disease patients' risk-benefit preferences: serious adverse event risks versus treatment efficacy. *Gastroenterology.* 2007;133(3):769-779.
8. Siegel CA, Levy L, Mackenzie T, Sands BE. Patient perceptions of the risks and benefits of infliximab. *Inflamm Bowel Dis.* 2008;14(1):1-6.
9. SEER. Surveillance, epidemiology, and ends results database. Available at: http://seer.cancer.gov. Accessed May 2, 2007.

SHOULD I MEASURE THIOPURINE METHYLTRANSFERASE GENOTYPE OR ENZYME ACTIVITY BEFORE STARTING A PATIENT ON AZATHIOPRINE OR 6-MERCAPTOPURINE?

Paul Rutgeerts, MD, PhD, FRCP; Gert Van Assche, MD, PhD; Séverine Vermeire, MD, PhD

Azathioprine or its metabolite 6-mercaptopurine (6-MP) are being used in Crohn's disease (CD) or ulcerative colitis (UC) for maintenance of remission and to avoid steroid use.[1,2] They are also used in the treatment of fistulizing CD and are recommended during episodic infliximab treatment to avoid antibody formation. Despite their proven efficacy, approximately 40% of inflammatory bowel disease (IBD) patients do not respond. Furthermore, 10% to 25% of patients have to withdraw azathioprine or 6-MP for major (leucopenia, pancreatitis, infection, and malignancy) or minor (rash, nausea, fever, arthralgias, headaches, malaise, and diarrhea) adverse events.[3,4] Myelosuppression is dose-dependent, can be lethal, and occurs in 1% to 5% of the patients.

Many factors will influence response and side effects to these drugs, including disease severity, concomitant medication, and genetic factors. Variability in drug response is greater across a population than within the same patient or in monozygotic twins. Therefore, part is attributed to genetic factors. It is estimated that polymorphisms in genes can account for 20% to 95% of variability in drug effects.[5]

Azathioprine is a pro-drug that is administered orally with highly variable gut absorption (16% to 50%). Azathioprine is degraded spontaneously to 6-MP and methylnitrothioimidazole. The further metabolism of 6-MP occurs through 3 competing enzymatic pathways, as outlined in Figure 8-1. One includes the conversion into 6-thioinosine monophosphate (6-TIMP) by the enzyme hypoxanthine-guanine phosphoribosyl

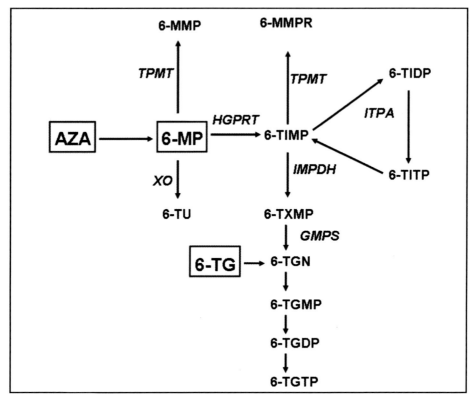

Figure 8-1. Azathioprine metabolism. Azathioprine is non-enzymatically converted to 6-MP. 6-MP is converted into the 6-thioinosine monophosphate (6-TIMP) by the enzyme hypoxanthine guanine phosphoribosyl-transferase (HGPRT). 6-TIMP is further metabolized to thioguanine mono-, di-, and triphosphates (6-thioguanine nucleotides [6-TGN]). Alternatively, 6-MP can be inactivated by xanthine oxidase (XO) or thiopurine methyltransferase (TPMT). TPMT also catalyses the methylation of the nucleotide metabolites, including 6-TIMP and 6-thioguanosine-5′-monophosphate (6-TGMP) to 6-methylmercaptopurine (6-MMPR). IMPDH = inosine monophosphate dehydrogenase; GMPS = guanine monophosphate synthetase; ITPA = inosine thriphosphare phyrophosphatase; 6-TITP = 6-thioinosine tryphosphare phyrophosphate.

transferase (HGPRT). 6-TIMP is then further metabolized to thioguanine mono-, di-, and triphosphates (thioguanine nucleotides, TGNs). Alternatively, 6-MP can be inactivated by xanthine oxidase (XO) into 6-thiouric acid (6-TU), or by thiopurine methyltransferase (TPMT) into 6-methylmercaptopurine (6-MMP). TPMT also catalyses the methylation of the nucleotide metabolites, including 6-TIMP and thioguanosine 5-monophosphate (TGMP).[6] The relative activities of the enzymes TPMT, XO, and HGPRT will determine the amount of the active 6-TGN and other 6-MP metabolites. The precise mechanism of action of the drug is not completely understood. The incorporation of TGNs in DNA plays a role in immune suppression and bone marrow toxicity.[7] More recent studies suggest that TGNs act by inhibition of Rac1 (Ras-related C3 botulinum toxin substrate 1), a guanosine triphosphate-binding (GTP) protein involved in the CD28 signal transduction pathway in T cells. CD28 co-stimulation is essential for T cell activation. Through inhibition of Rac1, its target genes (eg, mitogen-activated protein kinases, NF-κB, and bcl-x(L)) are suppressed.[8]

Twenty-five years ago, Weinshilboum et al described inherited differences in TPMT activity.[9] Since then, many variant alleles resulting in a decrease of enzymatic activity (TPMT*2, *3A, *3B, *3C, *3D, *4 through 15) have been described.[10-12] In the white and African populations, approximately 90% of individuals carry 2 wild-type alleles resulting in high TPMT enzyme activity; 10% are heterozygous and display intermediate activity; and 0.3% are homozygous for low activity alleles and display no detectable TPMT activity. Heterozygosity is less frequent in Asians (2% to 5%). The TPMT*2, *3A, and *3C alleles count for 80% to 95% of inherited TPMT deficiency in different populations over the world. The TPMT*2 allele contains a non-synonymous mutation at amino acid position 80 (Ala80Pro, G238C). The TPMT*3A allele contains 2 missense mutations, G460A (Ala145Thr) and A719G (Tyr240Cys). The TPMT*3C allele contains only the A719G missense mutation. In African, African-American, and Asian populations, the most common low TPMT activity allele is the TPMT*3C. In whites, it's the TPMT*3A allele.

Almost all patients who are heterozygous or homozygous for low-activity TPMT alleles develop severe hematotoxicity when treated with a normal thiopurine dose.[13-15] The inverse is not entirely true, as Colombel et al found that only 27% (11/41) of IBD patients who developed myelosuppression under azathioprine carried one or more TPMT variants.[16] However, in a study of patients treated with azathioprine for rheumatoid arthritis (RA), 5/6 patients (83%) with leucopenia were TPMT heterozygous.[17] The relationship between TPMT mutations, low TPMT enzyme activity, and myelosuppression with azathioprine is so straightforward that certain investigators suggest that thiopurine drugs should entirely be avoided, even in patients with low TPMT activity (heterozygous patients). It seems that the latter can mostly tolerate a reduced (50%) dose of azathioprine/6-MP, provided they are submitted to very close monitoring.[18,19] On the other hand, homozygous or compound heterozygous patients who will have almost absent TPMT activity should not receive the drug.

More recently, a relation between therapy refractoriness and normal or high TPMT activity has been described. Predicting response is equally useful, especially since there is a 3-month delay in onset of efficacy. Efficacy of treatment with 6-MP or azathioprine is related to red blood cell (RBC) levels of the active metabolite TGN (> 235 pmol/8x10*8 RBC).[15] Patients heterozygous for low TPMT activity alleles have lower TPMT activity and higher erythrocyte TGN levels.[20] One study showed a lower relapse rate in patients with low TPMT activity compared to patients with normal TPMT activity, but 2 later studies failed to replicate this finding.[20-22] High levels of 6-MMP are thought to be responsible for hepatotoxicity.[23] Liver transaminase elevation has been associated with high TPMT activity and 6-MMP levels, and TPMT variant alleles are very rare in patients with hepatotoxicity.

In clinical practice, genotyping the most common variants in the TPMT gene or measuring the enzyme activity are 2 alternative methods for predicting the risk for hematopoietic toxicity. Both techniques have advantages and disadvantages, so which to use will also depend on the availability in one's hospital. TPMT enzyme activity can be measured in RBCs with a radiochemical or high-performance liquid chromatography assay. However, the results can be influenced by recent blood transfusions, for instance.[24] TPMT activity also varies over time and is influenced by other drugs (eg, diuretics, 5-aminosalicyclic acid [5-ASA]) and conditions (eg, uremia).[25-27] TPMT enzyme activity will identify patients with high TPMT activity that metabolize 6-MP to 6-MMP and, therefore, may be resistant to treatment with thiopurine drugs.[23] Performing TPMT genotyping is done by polymerase chain reaction (PCR), and most will genotype only the most common variants here. However, over 30 variants in the gene have been described, but most are very rare. The correlation between the TPMT genotype and the enzyme activity is good, but not 100%. Patients with low to normal enzyme activity can have either a wild-type or a heterozygous genotype.[28] There is no consensus that TPMT genotype or phenotype should be measured before starting azathioprine or 6-MP treatment in IBD patients, especially since hematologic toxicity can develop in patients with normal TPMT activity. Monitoring blood counts and liver transaminases remains necessary in all patients. However, a socioeconomic study in IBD showed that TPMT phenotyping or genotyping is cost-effective to identify patients with low or no TPMT enzyme activity (homozygous or compound heterozygous) in order to not treat them and avoid severe hematological complications.[29] It is our standard clinical practice to perform TPMT genotyping in our patients before starting azathioprine. If TPMT enzyme activity is measured, patients with normal TPMT activity (or wild-type patients) can receive 2 to 2.5 mg/kg azathioprine or 1 to 1.5 mg/kg of 6-MP. Patients with intermediate activity (heterozygous) should have a dose reduction of 50%, and patients with low or absent TPMT activity (compound heterozygous or homozygous) should not receive thiopurine drugs at all.

References

1. Pearson DC, May GR, Fick G, Sutherland LR. Azathioprine for maintaining remission of Crohn's disease. *Cochrane Database Syst Rev.* 2000;(2):CD000067 [PM:10796482].
2. Sandborn W, Sutherland L, Pearson D, May G, Modigliani R, Prantera C. Azathioprine or 6-mercaptopurine for inducing remission of Crohn's disease. *Cochrane Database Syst Rev.* 2000;(2):CD000545 [PM:10796557].
3. Connell WR, Kamm MA, Ritchie JK, Lennard-Jones JE. Bone marrow toxicity caused by azathioprine in inflammatory bowel disease: 27 years of experience. *Gut.* 1993;34(8):1081-1085.
4. Present DH, Meltzer SJ, Krumholz MP, Wolke A, Korelitz BI. 6-Mercaptopurine in the management of inflammatory bowel disease: short- and long-term toxicity. *Ann Intern Med.* 1989;111(8):641-649.
5. Evans WE, McLeod HL. Pharmacogenomics—drug disposition, drug targets, and side effects. *N Engl J Med.* 2003;348(6):538-549.
6. Krynetski EY, Krynetskaia NF, Yanishevski Y, Evans WE. Methylation of mercaptopurine, thioguanine, and their nucleotide metabolites by heterologously expressed human thiopurine S-methyltransferase. *Mol Pharmacol.* 1995;47(6):1141-1147.
7. Lennard L. The clinical pharmacology of 6-mercaptopurine. *Eur J Clin Pharmacol.* 1992;43(4):329-339.
8. Tiede I, Fritz G, Strand S, et al. CD28-dependent Rac1 activation is the molecular target of azathioprine in primary human CD4+ T lymphocytes. *J Clin Invest.* 2003;111(8):1133-1145.
9. Weinshilboum RM, Sladek SL. Mercaptopurine pharmacogenetics: monogenic inheritance of erythrocyte thiopurine methyltransferase activity. *Am J Hum Genet.* 1980;32(5):651-662.
10. Evans WE. Pharmacogenetics of thiopurine S-methyltransferase and thiopurine therapy. *Ther Drug Monit.* 2004;26(2):186-191.
11. Alves S, Prata MJ, Ferreira F, Amorim A. Screening of thiopurine S-methyltransferase mutations by horizontal conformation-sensitive gel electrophoresis. *Hum Mutat.* 2000;15(3):246-253.
12. Lindqvist M, Haglund S, Almer S, et al. Identification of two novel sequence variants affecting thiopurine methyltransferase enzyme activity. *Pharmacogenetics.* 2004;14(4):261-265.
13. Gilissen LP, Derijks LJ, Bos LP, et al. Some cases demonstrating the clinical usefulness of therapeutic drug monitoring in thiopurine-treated inflammatory bowel disease patients. *Eur J Gastroenterol Hepatol.* 2004;16(7):705-710.
14. Ansari A, Hassan C, Duley J, et al. Thiopurine methyltransferase activity and the use of azathioprine in inflammatory bowel disease. *Aliment Pharmacol Ther.* 2002;16(10):1743-1750.
15. Cuffari C, Hunt S, Bayless T. Utilisation of erythrocyte 6-thioguanine metabolite levels to optimise azathioprine therapy in patients with inflammatory bowel disease. *Gut.* 2001;48(5):642-646.

16. Colombel JF, Ferrari N, Debuysere H, et al. Genotypic analysis of thiopurine S-methyltransferase in patients with Crohn's disease and severe myelosuppression during azathioprine therapy. *Gastroenterology.* 2000;118(6):1025-1030.
17. Black AJ, McLeod HL, Capell HA, et al. Thiopurine methyltransferase genotype predicts therapy-limiting severe toxicity from azathioprine. *Ann Intern Med.* 1998;129(9):716-718.
18. Seidman EG. Clinical use and practical application of TPMT enzyme and 6-mercaptopurine metabolite monitoring in IBD. *Rev Gastroenterol Disord.* 2003;3(suppl 1):S30-S38.
19. Kaskas BA, Louis E, Hindorf U, et al. Safe treatment of thiopurine S-methyltransferase deficient Crohn's disease patients with azathioprine. *Gut.* 2003;52(1):140-142.
20. Lowry PW, Franklin CL, Weaver AL, et al. Measurement of thiopurine methyltransferase activity and azathioprine metabolites in patients with inflammatory bowel disease. *Gut.* 2001;49(5):665-670.
21. Reuther LO, Sonne J, Larsen NE, et al. Pharmacological monitoring of azathioprine therapy. *Scand J Gastroenterol.* 2003;38(9):972-977.
22. Campbell S, Kingstone K, Ghosh S. Relevance of thiopurine methyltransferase activity in inflammatory bowel disease patients maintained on low-dose azathioprine. *Aliment Pharmacol Ther.* 2002;16(3):389-398.
23. Dubinsky MC, Yang H, Hassard PV, et al. 6-MP metabolite profiles provide a biochemical explanation for 6-MP resistance in patients with inflammatory bowel disease. *Gastroenterology.* 2002;122(4):904-915.
24. Schwab M, Schaeffeler E, Marx C, Zanger U, Aulitzky W, Eichelbaum M. Shortcoming in the diagnosis of TPMT deficiency in a patient with Crohn's disease using phenotyping only. *Gastroenterology.* 2001;121(2):498-499.
25. Lowry PW, Franklin CL, Weaver AL, et al. Leucopenia resulting from a drug interaction between azathioprine or 6-mercaptopurine and mesalamine, sulphasalazine, or balsalazide. *Gut.* 2001;49(5):656-664.
26. Giverhaug T, Klemetsdal B, Lysaa R, Aarbakke J. Intraindividual variability in red blood cell thiopurine methyltransferase activity. *Eur J Clin Pharmacol.* 1996;50(3):217-220.
27. Weyer N, Kroplin T, Fricke L, Iven H. Human thiopurine S-methyltransferase activity in uremia and after renal transplantation. *Eur J Clin Pharmacol.* 2001;57(2):129-136.
28. Spire-Vayron de la Moureyre C, Debuysere H, Mastain B, et al. Genotypic and phenotypic analysis of the polymorphic thiopurine S-methyltransferase gene (TPMT) in a European population. *Br J Pharmacol.* 1998;125(4):879-887.
29. Winter J, Walker A, Shapiro D, Gaffney D, Spooner RJ, Mills PR. Cost-effectiveness of thiopurine methyltransferase genotype screening in patients about to commence azathioprine therapy for treatment of inflammatory bowel disease. *Aliment Pharmacol Ther.* 2004;20(6):593-599.

HOW DO YOU MONITOR PATIENTS ON AZATHIOPRINE/6-MERCAPTOPURINE?

Miles Sparrow, MB, BS, FRACP

WHY MONITOR PATIENTS ON AZATHIOPRINE/ 6-MERCAPTOPURINE?

The thiopurine immunomodulators azathioprine and 6-mercaptopurine (6-MP) are well established as induction, maintenance, and steroid-sparing agents in the treatment of inflammatory bowel disease (IBD). All patients taking thiopurine immunomodulators require careful ongoing blood monitoring to detect potential adverse effects such as leukopenia or hepatotoxicity, and to avoid possible associated complications.

The primary aim of immunomodulator blood monitoring is to ensure treatment safety, but it also maximizes efficacy by helping avoid dose-dependent side effects that otherwise may lead to drug cessation. More recently, thiopurine metabolite measurements have added an additional means of optimizing immunodulator dosing, but they are complementary to, and in no way replace, routine blood monitoring.

WHAT TO MONITOR IN PATIENTS ON AZATHIOPRINE/ 6-MERCAPTOPURINE

You need to consider immunomodulator monitoring in 2 parts. The most important component of blood monitoring is the regular measurement of complete blood counts (CBC) and liver function tests (LFT), or so-called "routine bloods." The second part of monitoring, if necessary, involves measuring the thiopurine metabolites 6-thioguanine nucleotide (6-TGN) and 6-methylmercaptopurine (6-MMP).

WHEN AND HOW TO MONITOR PATIENTS ON AZATHIOPRINE/ 6-MERCAPTOPURINE

CBC AND LFT

The frequency of measuring these routine bloods depends on the duration of immunomodulator therapy, as outlined in Table 9-1.

- *How do you monitor CBC and LFT when starting therapy?*

    Leukopenia and hepatotoxicity most commonly, but not exclusively, occur soon after commencing thiopurines, or upon dose escalation. This means frequent blood monitoring is needed during the first 3 months of therapy. During the first 4 weeks, I recommend weekly CBC and LFT, followed by alternate weekly for the next 4 weeks, and then again at 12 weeks. This is a cautious approach aimed at detecting any leukopenia promptly and before infectious complications can occur. Thiopurine methyltransferase (TPMT) is an enzyme crucial to thiopurine metabolism, levels of which are approximately inversely proportional to the risk of developing leukopenia. If you are able to measure TPMT activity prior to commencing immunomodulator therapy and it is normal, then it is possible to reduce the frequency of initial testing to monthly, although routine bloods are definitely still necessary.

- *How do you monitor CBC and LFT when changing immunomodulator dose?*

    At any stage during therapy, if the thiopurine dose is increased, you need to check a CBC 2 weeks later to check for leukopenia, while dose reductions do not require monitoring blood tests. It is not necessary to check LFT with each dose escalation unless patients develop symptoms suggestive of hepatotoxicity, such as nausea.

- *How do you monitor CBC and LFT when patients are on a stable dose?*

    Leukopenia can occur at any time during thiopurine treatment. Therefore, CBC and LFT are required every 3 months for the duration of therapy. This is often overlooked, but one practical way of ensuring ongoing blood monitoring is to only give immunomodulator prescriptions for 3 months at a time.

- *What CBC and LFT blood results do you aim for?*

    The aim of therapy is immunomodulation without immunosuppression, and I aim for a total white cell count of greater than 3.5×10^9/L with a lymphocyte count greater than 1.0×10^9/L, or occasionally slightly lower. Asymptomatic elevations of hepatic transaminases only require dose reduction once they reach more than twice the upper limit of normal.

THIOPURINE METABOLITES

Historically, weight-based dosing of immunomodulators has been employed with target doses being 2.0 to 2.5 mg/kg for azathioprine and 1.0 to 1.5 mg/kg for 6-MP. More recently, advances in pharmacogenomics and an increased understanding of thiopurine metabolism has led to the practice of measuring TPMT enzyme activity prior to commencing therapy, and then using measurements of the thiopurine metabolites 6-TGN and 6-MMP to help optimize dosage and efficacy.

Azathioprine and 6-MP are both inactive pro-drugs that are metabolized by 3 competing enzymes, including TPMT, to produce the nucleotide metabolites 6-TGN and 6-MMP

Table 9-1
Blood Testing Monitoring Schedule for Azathioprine and 6-Mercaptopurine

Stage of Immunomodulator Therapy	Blood Monitoring Required
First month of therapy	Weekly
Second month of therapy	Alternate weekly
Third month of therapy	At 12 weeks
For the duration of therapy	3 monthly
After any dose escalation	2 weeks later

(Figure 9-1). TPMT activity within the population has a trimodal distribution with 89% of people possessing normal enzyme activity (homozygous high), 11% having intermediate activity (heterozygotes), and 0.3% having essentially no functional activity of the enzyme (homozygous low), with this last group being susceptible to prompt and potentially severe leukopenia on normal thiopurine doses. Retrospective studies, supported by meta-analyzed data, have shown that 6-TGN is the active metabolite responsible for the therapeutic efficacy and myelotoxicity of thiopurines, while 6-MMP levels have no correlation with efficacy, but instead are associated with hepatotoxicity when elevated. The 6-TGN metabolites appear to exert their immunomodulatory effects through several mechanisms, including via incorporating into lymphocytic DNA and inhibiting cellular replication, and also by way of the 6-TGN triphosphate moiety inducing apoptosis of activated lymphocytes. Numerically, 6-TGN levels of greater than 235 pmol/8 x 10^8 RBC correlate with an increased likelihood of response, while 6-MMP levels of greater than 5,700 pmol/8 x 10^8 RBC are associated with potentially dose-limiting hepatotoxicity.[1-3]

- *Do you need to measure TPMT prior to starting thiopurines?*

    Measuring TPMT prior to therapy allows you to identify the 1 in 300 patients deficient in the functional activity of the enzyme in whom these drugs should be avoided. This is very useful information, and it is recommended that if pharmacogenomic testing is available, it should be undertaken. However, if testing cannot be performed, then thiopurine therapy can still safely be commenced, provided careful blood monitoring is carried out as has been outlined.

- *When do you need to measure thiopurine metabolites?*

    Measuring the nucleotides 6-TGN and 6-MMP is only useful in patients who fail thiopurine treatment and who are unable to enter and maintain a steroid-free remission despite an adequate dose and duration of immunomodulator therapy. Conversely, if your patient is well and tolerating thiopurine therapy, then metabolite measurements do not provide any additional useful clinical information.

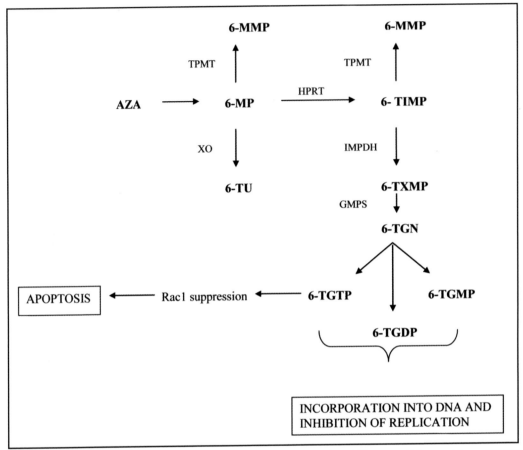

Figure 9-1. Metabolism of azathioprine and 6-mercaptopurine. XO = xanthine oxidase; TPMT = thiopurine methyltransferase; HPRT = hypoxanthine phosphoribosyltransferase; 6-TIMP = 6-thiosine 5'-monophosphate; IMPDH = inosine monophosphate dehydrogenase; GMPS = guanosine monophosphate synthetase; 6-TGMP = 6-thioguanine mono-phosphate; 6-TGDP = 6-thioguanine di-phosphate; 6-TGTP = 6-thioguanine tri-phosphate.

- *What do the results mean and how do we use them?*

  Measuring thiopurine metabolites effectively clarifies the reasons patients are not responding to immunomodulator therapy, and it identifies 4 groups of treatment failures (Table 9-2). The first group are patients with negligible or undetectable levels of both metabolites. These patients are likely to be noncompliant and can be questioned and managed accordingly. Confirming compliance before switching from thiopurine therapy is a justifiable reason for ordering metabolite testing. The second group are patients with low but detectable levels of both 6-TGN and 6-MMP. These patients are under-dosed and should tolerate dose escalation. The third group are patients with low 6-TGN levels and high 6-MMP levels. These patients have an unfavorable metabolite profile and are thiopurine "resistant." Further dose escalation is unlikely to be successful. The last group are patients with therapeutic, or high, levels of both 6-TGN and 6-MMP, and ongoing active disease. This group is truly thiopurine "refractory" and will require a different class of therapeutic agent.[4]

Table 9-2

Metabolite Profiles, Clinical Interpretations, and Management Recommendations for Thiopurine Treatment Non-Responders

	Metabolite Profile	Clinical Interpretation	Subsequent Management
Group 1	Negligible or undetectable 6-TGN and 6-MMP	Noncompliance	Confirmation and patient education
Group 2	Low 6-TGN; Low 6-MMP	Under-dosing	Dose escalation
Group 3	Low 6-TGN; High 6-MMP	Thiopurine "resistant"	Switch therapeutic class
Group 4	High 6-TGN; High 6-MMP	Thiopurine "refractory"	Switch therapeutic class

- *How often do you need to measure thiopurine metabolites?*

  The first set of metabolite measurements, which establishes the patient's genetically determined thiopurine metabolite profile, is the most important, and these can be performed after approximately 4 weeks of therapy. The confirmation of therapeutic metabolite levels by any subsequent dose adjustments should ideally be determined by a further set of metabolite levels 2 to 4 weeks later. Subsequent metabolite levels are thereafter only necessary if disease remission cannot be established or maintained at any time.

SUMMARY

Immunomodulator therapy with azathioprine and 6-MP is a cornerstone of IBD treatment, and it is used with the expectation of inducing and maintaining a corticosteroid-free remission in otherwise potentially refractory patients. The benefit-to-risk profile of these agents is usually favorable, provided they are used and monitored correctly. Routine blood testing for CBC and LFT is the most important component of monitoring to ensure the safety of these agents, and this is required for the entire duration a patient is taking thiopurine therapy. More recently, metabolite testing has provided additional information clarifying the reasons for an inadequate response to immunomodulators, therefore allowing for dosage optimization. However, this is complementary to and does not replace the need for ongoing routine blood monitoring.

References

1. Dubinsky MC, Lamothe S, Yang HY, et al. Pharmacogenomics and metabolite measurement for 6-mercapto-purine therapy in inflammatory bowel disease. *Gastroenterology.* 2000;118(4):705-713.
2. Osterman MT, Kundu R, Lichtenstein GR, Lewis, JD. Association of 6-thioguanine nucleotide levels and inflammatory bowel disease activity: a meta-analysis. *Gastroenterology.* 2006;130(4):1047-1053.
3. Tiede I, Fritz G, Strand S, et al. CD28-dependent Rac1 activation is the molecular target of azathioprine in primary human CD4+ T lymphocytes. *J Clin Invest.* 2003;111(8):1133-1145.
4. Gearry RB, Barclay ML. Azathioprine and 6-mercaptopurine pharmacogenetics and metabolite monitoring in inflammatory bowel disease. *J Gastroenterol Hepatol.* 2005;20(8):1149-1157.

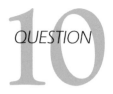

How Long Do You Wait Before Declaring Treatment Failure With Azathioprine/6-Mercaptopurine, and Do You Ever Consider Stopping Therapy With These Agents After a Period of Time?

Daniel H. Present, MD, MACG

Before you talk about treatment failure or withdrawing azathioprine/6-mercaptopurine (6-MP), the first question should be, "When do you use azathioprine/6-MP?" In my experience, you use it to induce and maintain remission in both Crohn's disease (CD) and ulcerative colitis (UC). In my many years of practice and clinical experience, these agents are the most effective therapy we have for treating inflammatory bowel disease (IBD). The "long-term" clinical response is greater than that seen with biologics. In CD, 6-MP is not only effective in inducing clinical response and remission in about three-quarters of patients, but it also has demonstrated the ability to maintain the response long-term (over 4 years). Azathioprine and 6-MP have shown endoscopic mucosal healing, and in one study, they have been effective in preventing postoperative recurrence after resection of CD.[1,2]

In the more recent studies, 6-MP and azathioprine have been shown to prevent antibody formation when biologicals are administered in an on-demand regimen.[1]

Of great importance is the ability of 6-MP and azathioprine to heal fistulas (both internal and external) in about one-third of patients. Another one-third of patients will show improvement in fistula symptoms. In my experience, I believe it is an error to start biologicals before a trial of 6-MP/azathioprine.[2,3]

It has been said that these agents take too long for response, but, in fact, within 2 months, 56% of the patients who are going to respond will have done so. At 3 months, almost 70% of those patients who are going to respond have done so. CD is a disease of a lifetime, and in many patients, there is no rush to institute steroids or biologicals. Instead, it is prudent to wait for the response to 6-MP/azathioprine.[3]

Although used to a lesser degree, it has also been clearly shown that 6-MP and azathioprine are effective in UC. In both uncontrolled and controlled data, azathioprine is effective in both inducing and maintaining a remission. A recent study has shown that azathioprine will allow complete steroid sparing in 53% of patients, whereas 5-aminosalicyclic acid (5-ASA) drugs are effective in only 21% after steroids are initiated. In my clinical experience, 6-MP will prevent colectomy in about one-third of patients in whom surgery is being considered.[4]

The ability to maintain response in both CD and UC answers the second part of the question: "Do I ever consider stopping therapy with these agents after a period of time?" I now have patients who have been taking this drug for 25 years. In my practice, I have not seen an increased risk of atypical infections, nor have I seen an increased risk of neoplasia (both carcinoma and lymphoma). I advise my patients to stay on the drug "forever," or until we physicians become smarter. A prospective double-blind withdrawal study should be considered in patients who have been in remission for 10 years or longer and who have demonstrated complete mucosal healing.

Going back to the first question, I noted that the mean time to respond is approximately 3 months. However, I have had a subgroup of patients respond after 6 months. In controlled trials, the mean dose of 6-MP to respond is only 75 mg daily. If there has been no evidence of response at 3 to 4 months, I then raise the dose to 100 mg. If there is still no response, I will go up to 150 mg. If this is ineffective, then the patient probably has excess thiopurine methyltransferase (TPMT). In that situation, 6-MP would normally have to be stopped. However, recent studies using allopurinol to block excess TPMT have shown success in steroid-sparing and clinical response. If allopurinol is ineffective, then consideration should be given to switching to methotrexate (MTX) in CD and perhaps a biological in UC.[3]

In summary, start 6-MP or azathioprine early in the course, maintain it, and do not give up on the drug until at least 5 to 6 months. When responding, maintain the agent long-term. I tell patients that until we have better agents, both diamonds and 6-MP/azathioprine are forever.

References

1. Velayos F, Mahadevan U. Management of steroid-dependant ulcerative colitis: immunomodulatory agents, biologics, or surgery? *Clin Gastroenterol Hepatol.* 2007;5(6):668-671.
2. Sandborn WJ, Feagan BG, Lichtenstein GR. Medical management of mild to moderate Crohn's disease: evidence-based treatment algorithms for induction and maintenance of remission. *Aliment Pharmacol Ther.* 2007;26(7):987-1003.
3. Present DH. Interaction of 6-mercaptopurine and azathioprine with 5-aminosalicylic acid agents. *Gastroenterology.* 2000;119(1):276.
4. Ardizzone S, Maconi G, Russo A, Imbesi V, Colombo E, Bianchi Porro G. Randomized controlled trial of azathioprine and 5-aminosalicylic acid for treatment of steroid dependent ulcerative colitis. *Gut.* 2006;55(1):47-53.

11

MY PARTNER USES METHOTREXATE AS HIS FIRST LINE AGENT IN CROHN'S DISEASE. HOW DO YOU CHOOSE BETWEEN 6-MERCAPTOPURINE AND METHOTREXATE?

A. Hillary Steinhart, MD, MSc, FRCPC

When one is deciding between using a purine antimetabolite (azathioprine and 6-mercaptopurine [6-MP]) or methotrexate (MTX) for the treatment of patients with Crohn's disease (CD), it is helpful to first examine what we know about the efficacy of the 2 classes of agents. There have been controlled trials of both classes of medication that have demonstrated their efficacy when compared to placebo, but there has only been one trial that has directly compared azathioprine/6-MP with that of MTX.[1] Although that study provides only limited information regarding the relative benefits of the 2 therapies, there are certain characteristics that can permit one to choose between them.

ONSET OF ACTION

Azathioprine/6-MP is known to have a relatively slow onset of maximal action (approximately 3 to 4 months on average), whereas MTX has a somewhat faster onset of action, with clinical efficacy seen within as little as 6 weeks.[2] This reported difference in the onset of action may be one reason to choose one therapy over the other. For example, if a patient has symptoms due to active disease and is on no other means of effective induction therapy, there is usually a need for a therapy that provides a faster response or faster reduction in symptoms. In that instance, MTX may be the preferred agent because of the more rapid onset of action. However, if a patient has been placed on an acute induction course of steroids, then azathioprine/6-MP may the more appropriate choice for its demonstrated steroid-sparing effect and its ability to maintain remission induced by steroids.[3,4] Azathioprine/6-MP has not been shown to be effective in trials where the duration of therapy was less than 4 months or where an acute treatment effect (ie, induction of remission) was the outcome of interest.[5,6] However, the North American Crohn's Study Group demonstrated that MTX is effective by 16 weeks of treatment at bringing chronically active steroid refractory CD into clinical remission and allowing steroid tapering.[2] In that study, the proportion of patients in remission and off steroids after 16 weeks of 25 mg of intramuscular (IM) MTX was approximately 40%, which was roughly twice the proportion in the placebo-treated patients. In addition, a significant treatment response was seen by 6 weeks of MTX therapy. Although not directly comparable because of differences in patient populations, the likelihood of a patient being in remission and remaining off of steroids more than 6 months after having been placed on maintenance doses of azathioprine or 6-MP is approximately twice that of a patient not receiving azathioprine/6-MP.[7]

An Italian study attempted to compare the use of azathioprine and MTX in an investigator-blinded trial.[1] MTX was given intravenously for 3 months and then orally thereafter, and all of the patients received an induction course of corticosteroids. Although the investigators concluded that there was no difference in the rapidity of the onset of action, the use of an induction course of steroids could have obscured any potential difference between the 2 groups.

References

1. Ardizzone S, Bollani S, Manzionna G, Imbesi V, Colombo E, Bianchi PG. Comparison between methotrexate and azathioprine in the treatment of chronic active Crohn's disease: a randomized, investigator-blind study. *Dig Liver Dis.* 2003;35(9):619-627.
2. Feagan BG, Rochon J, Fedorak RN, et al. Methotrexate for the treatment of Crohn's disease. The North American Crohn's Study Group Investigators. *N Engl J Med.* 1995;332(5):292-297.
3. Candy S, Wright J, Gerber M, Adams G, Gerig M, Goodman R. A controlled double-blind study of azathioprine in the management of Crohn's disease. *Gut.* 1995;37(5):674-678.
4. Markowitz J, Grancher K, Kohn N, Lesser M, Daum F. A multicenter trial of 6-mercaptopurine and prednisone in children with newly diagnosed Crohn's disease. *Gastroenterology.* 2000;119(4):895-902.
5. Present DH, Korelitz BI, Wisch N, Glass JL, Sachar DB, Pasternack BS. Treatment of Crohn's disease with 6-mercaptopurine. A long-term, randomized, double-blind study. *N Engl J Med.* 1980;302(18):981-987.
6. Summers RW, Switz DM, Sessions JT Jr, et al. National cooperative Crohn's disease study: results of drug treatment. *Gastroenterology.* 1979;77(4 pt 2):847-869.
7. Pearson DC, May GR, Fick G, Sutherland LR. Azathioprine for maintaining remission of Crohn's disease. *The Cochrane Library Issue 1.* 2000. Oxford, Update Software.

If I Want to Use Methotrexate for My Patients With Crohn's Disease, What Dose(s) and What Route of Administration (Subcutaneous, Intramuscular, or Oral) Should I Use? Is There a Risk of Hepatotoxicity or Pulmonary Toxicity?

A. Hillary Steinhart, MD, MSc, FRCPC

Following induction therapy with methotrexate (MTX) 25 mg intramuscular (IM) weekly, further MTX given at a dose of 15 mg IM once weekly has been shown to maintain remission and reduce steroid requirements in Crohn's disease (CD).[1] In general, subcutaneous (SC) dosing can be given instead of IM, and, for some patients with normal small intestinal absorptive function, oral (per os; PO) dosing can be given.

CONVENIENCE, TOLERABILITY, AND ADVERSE EVENT PROFILE

If 2 therapies are roughly equivalent with respect to their ability to reduce symptoms, maintain remission, and reduce steroid requirements, then their convenience, safety, and tolerability become relatively more important in deciding which to use. Both azathioprine/6-mercaptopurine (6-MP) and MTX have been used for many years, and most clinicians treating patients with inflammatory bowel disease (IBD) are familiar with their potential side effects. (See Question 8 on page 33 and Question 9 on page 39 for dosing and monitoring of azathioprine/6-MP.)

Although MTX has been studied primarily when given by the IM route, absorption of MTX is equally good when given by SC injection. This has the advantage of allowing patient self-administration, but it may still be an obstacle for some patients. In some cases, MTX is given in combination with infliximab in order to reduce immunogenicity and the formation of antibodies against infliximab. The dose of MTX required to produce this effect is not precisely known, but it may be lower than the usual maintenance dose. At a dose of less than 15 mg weekly, the absorption of PO administered MTX is more consistent than it is at higher doses, thereby allowing PO administration when low doses are used.

The most common side effects associated with MTX use are anorexia, nausea, vomiting, and diarrhea. It is thought that the frequency of these side effects, which may be as high as 50%, can be reduced or the symptoms can be ameliorated by the administration of folic acid at least 2 days removed from the weekly MTX dose.

The risk of bone marrow suppression with the doses of MTX generally used for the treatment of CD is low, but regular monitoring of complete blood count (CBC) is still required. The frequency of monitoring is generally every 2 weeks for the first month, and then every 2 to 3 months thereafter. The risk of bone marrow suppression may also be reduced by folic acid administration.

Liver enzyme (serum transaminase) abnormalities have been reported in up to 30% of patients in some series. When enzyme elevations are below 2 times the upper limit of normal, they generally require no change in therapy or only temporary dosage reduction. Intermittent liver enzyme abnormalities may indicate an increased risk of hepatic fibrosis with ongoing MTX use. It appears that the risk of fibrosis is extremely low when there has been no liver enzyme abnormality throughout the course of MTX therapy. Routine liver biopsies to monitor for fibrosis are not recommended for IBD patients on MTX.[2] However, considering a liver biopsy after a cumulative dose of 4 g is prudent in patients who have had frequent elevations of their serum transaminases.

Pulmonary toxicity rarely occurs, but it can be serious. It is typically a hypersensitivity pneumonitis and should be suspected when a patient on MTX develops fever, cough, dyspnea, or chest pain, often with pulmonary infiltrate on a chest x-ray. Bronchoalveolar lavage can help confirm the diagnosis, and MTX discontinuation is required. Steroid treatment can be used in patients not improving after discontinuation or who are seriously ill.

References

1. Feagan BG, Fedorak RN, Irvine EJ, et al. A comparison of methotrexate with placebo for the maintenance of remission in Crohn's disease. North American Crohn's Study Group Investigators. *N Engl J Med.* 2000;342(22):1627-1632.
2. Te HS, Schiano TD, Kuan SF, Hanauer SB, Conjeevaram HS, Baker AL. Hepatic effects of long-term methotrexate use in the treatment of inflammatory bowel disease. *Am J Gastroenterol.* 2000;95(11):3150-3156.

WHICH PATIENTS MIGHT BE BETTER FOR A "TOP-DOWN" APPROACH (USING ANTI-TUMOR NECROSIS FACTOR THERAPY BEFORE STEROIDS OR PROVEN FAILURE OF ORAL THIOPURINES)? WHAT CLINICAL BEHAVIOR OR SEROLOGICAL MARKERS MIGHT YOU USE TO IDENTIFY THESE PATIENTS?

Sonia Friedman, MD

"Top-down versus step-up therapy" is a catchy phrase, and in a era where mucosal healing is becoming more and more important, it might seem attractive to initiate an anti-tumor necrosis factor (TNF) drug as the initial therapy for Crohn's disease (CD). In rheumatoid arthritis (RA), anti-TNF agents are started early and given aggressively, often in combination with an immunomodulator such as methotrexate (MTX). For RA patients, anti-TNF therapies have prevented irreversible and debilitating destruction of the affected joints. But is the data in CD comparable to the data in RA? Should the inflamed and ulcerated gut be treated the same way as inflamed and deformed joints?

In the single study comparing "step-up" with "top-down" therapy in CD, 133 steroid-, immunomodulator-, and biologic-naïve patients with moderate to severe disease were randomized to receive either steroids (methylprednisolone or budesonide) or 3 induction doses of infliximab + maintenance azathioprine (2 to 2.5 mg/kg/day). Patients were given MTX if they were unable to take azathioprine. Patients in the steroid group "stepped up" to azathioprine, and then 3 induction doses of infliximab, if needed. The endpoints of the study were remission determined by a Crohn's Disease Activity Index (CDAI) score of < 150 off of steroids, and avoidance of bowel resection at 26 and 52 weeks.[1]

The results here were impressive. At 26 weeks, 60% of patients in the infliximab + azathioprine group were in remission, off of steroids, and without surgical resection, versus 35.9% in the conventional treatment. At 52 weeks, the figures were 61.5% versus 42.2%, respectively (Figure 13-1). Patients in the infliximab + azathioprine group also had significantly better mucosal healing at colonoscopy (Figure 13-2). There was no difference in adverse events between the 2 groups. At 52 weeks, almost 100% of patients were on either azathioprine or MTX versus 73% in the conventional group.

Should we be giving every Crohn's patient who has failed 5-aminosalicyclic acid (5-ASA) agents and antibiotics 3 induction doses of infliximab? If therapeutic doses of azathioprine had been started with the steroids, would the results of this study be different? Would mucosal healing still have been achieved? There is not yet a study that answers these specific questions.

Another recent study looked at the induction of remission in patients with steroid-dependent CD. These patients had been on prednisone for at least 6 months, and despite this, still had active disease. Doses of prednisone ranged from 20 to 46 mg/day. The study group consisted of both 6-mercaptopurine- (6-MP) and azathioprine-naïve patients and patients who had been on stable doses of one of these medications for at least 6 months. Patients received 3 induction doses of infliximab + 6-MP/azathioprine or placebo + 6-MP/azathioprine and were followed for up to 52 weeks. Results were not surprising, as patients on infliximab did better than those on placebo. Since patients only got 3 infusions, the effect of infliximab was gradually diminished over a year. At week 52, infliximab was more effective as a "bridge" therapy in patients who had been 6-MP/azathioprine-naïve versus those who had been 6-MP/azathioprine failures (52% versus 27% clinical remission off of steroids). In addition, mucosal healing was significantly better in the infliximab group. Patients who were naïve to 6-MP/azathioprine also did better with placebo than those who had previously failed 6-MP/azathioprine (32% versus 12% clinical remission off of steroids).[2]

Although these are results from a steroid-dependent group of Crohn's patients, several lessons apply. First, infliximab can be effective when steroids alone or in combination with 6-MP/azathioprine fail. Second, although infliximab + 6-MP/azathioprine is more effective than 6-MP/azathioprine alone, 6-MP and azathioprine are still highly effective drugs. No doses of 6-MP/azathioprine and no thiopurine metabolite levels were given in this paper, so we really don't know whether these drugs reached therapeutic levels. In other studies, 6-MP/azathioprine have up to a 60% remission rate in steroid-dependent CD. In the ACCENT 1 (A Crohn's Disease Clinical Trial Evaluating Infliximab in a New Long-Term Treatment Regimen) study, at 30 weeks, the highest remission rate was 45% for patients receiving infusions of infliximab every 8 weeks. Third, there have been no head-to-head trials of infliximab versus 6-MP/azathioprine versus infliximab + 6-MP/azathioprine that have yet been published, so we really don't know which is more effective in patients who are steroid-naïve. A SONIC (Study of Immunomodulatory-Naïve Patients in Crohn's Disease) presentation that has not yet been published in a peer-reviewed journal looked at this question and indicated that infliximab + azathioprine may be the most effective induction therapy for patients with moderate to severe CD who may or may not be steroid-naïve.[3]

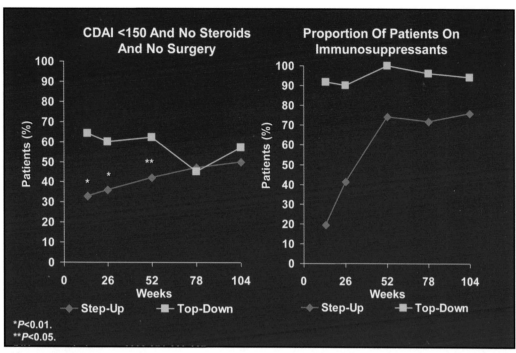

Figure 13-1. Results of a top-down versus a step-up approach. Reproduced with permission from *Current Perspectives on Treatment and Management of Crohn's Disease* CME lecture series sponsored by PIM and VIM.

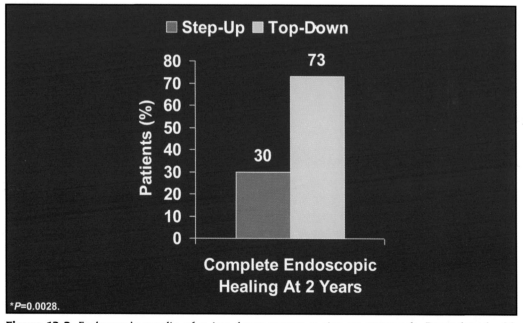

Figure 13-2. Endoscopic results of a top-down versus a step-up approach. Reproduced with permission from *Current Perspectives on Treatment and Management of Crohn's Disease* CME lecture series sponsored by PIM and VIM.

If infliximab is more effective than 6-MP/azathioprine, is it safe enough for widespread use as the primary therapy for CD? In the Mayo Clinic series of 500 patients, there were 5 deaths attributable to infliximab—two due to sepsis, and 3 due to malignancies.[4] In addition, there have been 12 case reports of the rare hepatosplenic T cell lymphoma (HSTCL) in patients on infliximab and immunomodulators.[5] With the recent advent of thiopurine methyltransferase (TPMT) phenotyping, 6-MP/azathioprine can be aggressively dosed, and results can often be seen at 4 to 6 weeks. Even if we wait the full 3 to 4 months for these drugs to take effect, this is a short time period in the life of a Crohn's patient. In general, nothing irrevocable is going to happen in 3 to 4 months that would preclude use or benefit of the anti-TNF therapies. We even have tricks now to make 6-MP/azathioprine work better, such as monitoring 6-thioguanine (6-TG)/6-methylmercaptopurine (6-MMP) levels and using allopurinol in patients who preferentially metabolize to the 6-MMP pathway.

There are a few groups of patients, however, who do benefit from primary anti-TNF therapy. Recently published predictors of disabling CD included an initial requirement for steroid use, an age below 40 years, and a perianal disease at initial diagnosis.[6] I believe that patients with severe perianal fistulizing disease deserve prompt anti-TNF therapy because this condition can be debilitating, the thiopurines take longer to work, and they are probably not as effective. Patients with severe colitis, deep ulcerations, and systemic symptoms should be treated initially with anti-TNF therapy. Patients with rectovaginal fistulas should be treated initially with anti-TNF therapy because 6-MP/azathioprine have a lower likelihood of working in this setting. Patients with ileo-anal J pouches who were initially thought to have ulcerative colitis (UC) and then develop a pouch fistula many years after surgery should be treated aggressively with anti-TNF therapy. Lastly, patients who have trouble absorbing oral medications, such as those with short bowel syndrome, should be treated with parenteral medications. Anti-TNF therapy and MTX may both be appropriate in this setting.

Although Serology 7 profiles have now been shown to identify certain groups with CD at a high risk for complications, I do not believe that they are helpful in determining whether a patient should be placed on anti-TNF therapy rather than aggressively dosed on 6-MP/azathioprine. Given the general lack of efficacy of 5-ASA medications in CD, the lack of mucosal healing, and the severe side effects of steroids, most patients with moderate to severe disease should be placed on 6-MP/azathioprine or MTX when appropriate. At this point in time, Serology 7 does not trump clinical evaluation when picking out the most severe patients who need primary anti-TNF therapy.

There are many new therapies for CD, both in current use and on the horizon. We have seen much success with infliximab, adalimumab, certolizumab, and natalizumab, but we have also seen adverse side effects. We have 50 years of experience with 6-MP/azathioprine in CD and only 11 years since the first infliximab clinical trial was published. We now have the ability to measure 6-MP/azathioprine phenotype and metabolites. Although expensive, these tests have the ability to better guide thiopurine therapy. With a few exceptions, I think most patients deserve a trial of therapeutically dosed 6-MP/azathioprine, and in many cases, MTX, before "stepping up" to anti-TNF therapy.

References

1. D'Haens G, Baert F, van Assche G, et al. Early combined immunosuppression or conventional management in patients with newly diagnosed Crohn's disease: an open randomized trial. *Lancet.* 2008;371(9613):660-667.
2. Lemann M, Mary JY, Duclos B, et al. Infliximab plus azathioprine for steroid-dependent Crohn's disease patients: a randomized placebo-controlled trial. *Gastroenterology.* 2006;130(4):1054-1061.
3. Sandborn W, Rutgeerts P, Reinisch W, et al. A randomized, double-blind, controlled trial comparing infliximab and infliximab plus azathioprine to azathioprine in patients with Crohn's disease naïve to immunomodulators and biologic therapy: the SONIC trial. *Am J Gastroenterol.* ACG 2008.
4. Columbel JF, Loftus EV, Tremaine WJ, et al. The safety profile of infliximab in patients with Crohn's disease: the Mayo Clinic experience in 500 patients. *Gastroenterology.* 2004;126(1):19-31.
5. Mackey AC, Green L, Liang LC, et al. Hepatosplenic T cell lymphoma associated with infliximab use in young patients treated for inflammatory bowel disease. *J Pediatric Gastroenterol Nutr.* 2007;44(2):265-267.
6. Beaugerie L, Seksik P, Nion-Larmurier I, et al. Predictors of Crohn's disease. *Gastroenterology.* 2006;130(3):650-656.

How Do You Approach Polypoid Lesions in Patients with Inflammatory Bowel Disease?

Francis A. Farraye, MD, MSc, FACG, FASGE

Patients with long-standing ulcerative colitis (UC) are at an increased risk for developing dysplasia and colorectal carcinoma (CRC). This risk approaches 8% by 20 years, and 18% by 30 years.[1] More recent data suggests that the risk of CRC in patients with UC may be lower than previously reported.[2,3] Patients with extensive Crohn's colitis also have an increased risk of CRC and should undergo regular surveillance.[4] At present, despite a lack of evidence from randomized controlled trials,[5] surveillance colonoscopy is the best and most widely used method to detect dysplasia and cancer in inflammatory bowel disease (IBD) patients.[6-9] However, there are several limitations to surveillance colonoscopy and colonoscopy practices that are not uniform.[10] Multiple biopsies are needed, which is time-consuming. It has been estimated that 33 biopsies are needed to achieve 90% confidence to detect dysplasia if it is present.[11] Colonoscopic biopsies should be characterized pathologically as negative, indefinite for dysplasia, or positive for low-grade dysplasia (LGD), high-grade dysplasia (HGD), or carcinoma.[12] There are only moderate levels of agreement among pathologists on the diagnosis of dysplasia with better agreement for HGD versus negative than LGD versus indefinite. An expert gastrointestinal (GI) pathologist should confirm all cases of dysplasia. Of utmost importance, the success of any surveillance program depends on patient compliance with regular colonoscopy.

Dysplasia in IBD may occur in flat mucosa (endoscopically invisible) or as an elevated lesion on endoscopy. The finding of flat HGD or carcinoma (confirmed by 2 expert GI pathologists) in endoscopic biopsy samples is an indication for colectomy.[13] There is accumulating evidence to suggest that flat LGD is also an indication for colectomy because of the relatively high rate of progression to HGD or cancer.[3,13-15] The approach to the patient with flat dysplasia is discussed in Question 16 on page 67.

Recent studies by Rutter and Rubin suggest that most dysplasia found in patients with IBD is elevated.[16,17] Blackstone and colleagues first described the term DALM (dysplasia-associated lesion or mass) in 1981. In Blackstone's study of 12 patients with DALMs, 7 were malignant,[18] and, consequently, any raised dysplastic lesion was felt to be an indication for colectomy. However, it is now apparent that DALMs actually represent a heterogeneous population of tumors in which the cancer risk is not equal among these various subtypes. Raised dysplastic lesions with the appearance of sporadic adenomas have been termed adenoma-like DALMs.[19] Adenoma-like DALMs are well circumscribed, sessile, or pedunculated lesions without hemorrhage, ulceration, or necrosis that resemble sporadic adenomas in patients who do not have IBD (Figure 14-1). In contrast, non–adenoma-like DALMs are defined as irregular, broad-based, or poorly circumscribed lesions that often contain foci of ulceration, necrosis, or hemorrhage (Figure 14-2). Inflammatory polyps have a typical endoscopic appearance (typically small, multiple, glistening, and filiform), have no malignant potential, and, thus, do not mandate removal (Figure 14-3 A, B).

Several reports have described the conservative management of small polypoid dysplastic lesions in patients with IBD. Recent studies have demonstrated that patients with adenoma-like DALMs may be treated adequately by polypectomy and continued surveillance because of their low association with cancer. However, non–adenoma-like DALMs still remain an indication for colectomy because of their high association with cancer.[20-23] In one study, polypoid dysplastic lesions with the appearance of adenomas could be identified and removed by standard endoscopic techniques. In the absence of flat dysplasia surrounding the lesion or elsewhere in the colon, the risk of the development of dysplasia or colorectal cancer was low over an 82-month follow-up period.[21] Rubin and colleagues demonstrated similar results in a cohort of patients followed for a mean of 49 months.[22] Close follow-up endoscopic surveillance is required for patients in which a polypoid dysplastic lesion is removed. In general, the initial surveillance colonoscopy is in 3 months, and if no dysplasia is identified, the next procedure can be in 12 months.

If a dysplastic-appearing polyp is encountered (Figure 14-4) and felt to be endoscopically amenable to resection, it should be removed by standard snare cautery techniques. Additional biopsies need to be taken around the polypectomy site as well as throughout the colon. Dysplastic polyps located proximal to an area of colitis can be managed as a sporadic adenoma. Finally, classic-appearing pseudopolyps do not require endoscopic resection or biopsy, though there should be a low threshold to do so if there are any atypical features present. A recent internet-based study determined that academic and private practice gastroenterologists have more difficulty than IBD experts in distinguishing between and managing polypoid dysplastic lesions in patients with UC.[24]

Newer techniques are needed to facilitate the identification of neoplastic lesions in patients with IBD. Chromoendoscopy may be the technique most readily applicable in clinical practice.[25,26] Chromoendoscopy can improve the detection of subtle colonic lesions, raising the sensitivity of the endoscopic examination, and it can improve lesion characterization, increasing the specificity of the examination. Additionally, crypt architecture can be categorized using the pit pattern, aiding differentiation between neoplastic and non-neoplastic changes, and enabling the performance of targeted biopsies. Several different stains have been used, including contrast stains (indigo carmine) and vital stains (methylene blue). We await additional studies to determine if chromoendoscopy with targeted biopsies will replace our standard procedure of multiple random biopsies. Finally, a recent study demonstrated that confocal chromoscopic endomicroscopy was superior to standard chromoendoscopy with methylene blue for the detection of dysplasia in patients with UC.[27]

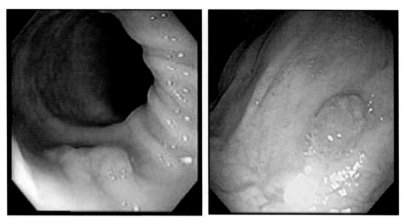

Figure 14-1. Adenoma-like DALM.

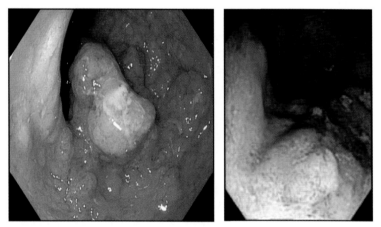

Figure 14-2. Non–adenoma-like DALM.

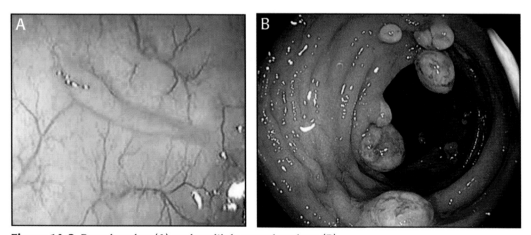

Figure 14-3. Pseudopolyp (A) and multiple pseudopolyps (B).

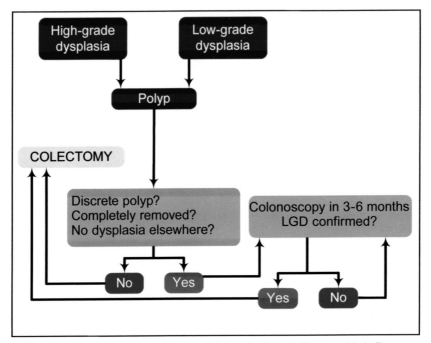

Figure 14-4. Management of polypoid dysplasia in patients with inflammatory bowel disease. Reprinted from *Gastroenterology*, 126(6), Itzkowitz SH, Harpaz N, Diagnosis and management of dysplasia in patients with inflammatory bowel diseases, 1634-1648, Copyright 2004, with permission from Elsevier.

In summary, dysplasia in patients with IBD may be flat or polypoid. Polypoid dysplasia that is completely excised and unassociated with flat dysplasia surrounding the polyp or elsewhere in the colon can be managed by polypectomy alone and continued surveillance.

References

1. Eaden J. Review article: colorectal carcinoma and inflammatory bowel disease. *Aliment Pharmacol Ther.* 2004;20(suppl 4):24-30.
2. Loftus EV Jr. Epidemiology and risk factors for colorectal dysplasia and cancer in ulcerative colitis. *Gastroenterol Clin North Am.* 2006;35(3):517-531.
3. Rutter MD, Saunders BP, Wilkinson KH, et al. Thirty-year analysis of a colonoscopic surveillance program for neoplasia in ulcerative colitis. *Gastroenterology.* 2006;130(4):1030-1038.
4. Friedman S, Rubin PH, Bodian C, Goldstein E, Harpaz N, Present DH. Screening and surveillance colonoscopy in chronic Crohn's colitis. *Gastroenterology.* 2001;120(4):820-826.
5. Collins PD, Mpofu C, Watson AJ, Rhodes JM. Strategies for detecting colon cancer and/or dysplasia in patients with inflammatory bowel disease. *Cochrane Database Syst Rev.* 2006(2):CD000279.
6. Itzkowitz SH, Present DH. Consensus conference: Colorectal cancer screening and surveillance in inflammatory bowel disease. *Inflamm Bowel Dis.* 2005;11(3):314-321.
7. Itzkowitz SH, Harpaz N. Diagnosis and management of dysplasia in patients with inflammatory bowel diseases. *Gastroenterology.* 2004;126(6):1634-1648.
8. Eaden JA, Mayberry JF. Guidelines for screening and surveillance of asymptomatic colorectal cancer in patients with inflammatory bowel disease. *Gut.* 2002;51(suppl 5):V10-12.

9. Winawer S, Fletcher R, Rex D, et al. Colorectal cancer screening and surveillance: clinical guidelines and rationale-Update based on new evidence. *Gastroenterology.* 2003;124(2):544-560.

10. Rodriguez SA, Eisen GM. Surveillance and management of dysplasia in ulcerative colitis by US gastroenterologists: in truth, a good performance. *Gastrointest Endosc.* 2007;66(5):1070.

11. Rubin CE, Haggitt RC, Burmer GC, et al. DNA aneuploidy in colonic biopsies predicts future development of dysplasia in ulcerative colitis. *Gastroenterology.* 1992;103(5):1611-1620.

12. Riddell RH, Goldman H, Ransohoff DF, et al. Dysplasia in inflammatory bowel disease: standardized classification with provisional clinical applications. *Hum Pathol.* 1983;14(11):931-968.

13. Bernstein CN, Shanahan F, Weinstein WM. Are we telling patients the truth about surveillance colonoscopy in ulcerative colitis? *Lancet.* 1994;343(8889):71-74.

14. Thomas T, Abrams KA, Robinson RJ, Mayberry JF. Meta-analysis: cancer risk of low-grade dysplasia in chronic ulcerative colitis. *Aliment Pharmacol Ther.* 2007;25(6):657-668.

15. Ullman T, Croog V, Harpaz N, Sachar D, Itzkowitz S. Progression of flat low-grade dysplasia to advanced neoplasia in patients with ulcerative colitis. *Gastroenterology.* 2003;125(5):1311-1319.

16. Rubin DT, Rothe JA, Hetzel JT, Cohen RD, Hanauer SB. Are dysplasia and colorectal cancer endoscopically visible in patients with ulcerative colitis? *Gastrointest Endosc.* 2007;65(7):998-1004.

17. Rutter MD, Saunders BP, Wilkinson KH, Kamm MA, Williams CB, Forbes A. Most dysplasia in ulcerative colitis is visible at colonoscopy. *Gastrointest Endosc.* 2004;60(3):334-339.

18. Blackstone MO, Riddell RH, Rogers BH, Levin B. Dysplasia-associated lesion or mass (DALM) detected by colonoscopy in long-standing ulcerative colitis: an indication for colectomy. *Gastroenterology.* 1981;80(2):366-374.

19. Odze RD. Adenomas and adenoma-like DALMs in chronic ulcerative colitis: a clinical, pathological, and molecular review. *Am J Gastroenterol.* 1999;94(7):1746-1750.

20. Engelsgjerd M, Farraye FA, Odze RD. Polypectomy may be adequate treatment for adenoma-like dysplastic lesions in chronic ulcerative colitis. *Gastroenterology.* 1999;117(6):1288-94.

21. Odze RD, Farraye FA, Hecht JL, Hornick JL. Long-term follow-up after polypectomy treatment for adenoma-like dysplastic lesions in ulcerative colitis. *Clin Gastroenterol Hepatol.* 2004;2(7):534-541.

22. Rubin PH, Friedman S, Harpaz N, et al. Colonoscopic polypectomy in chronic colitis: conservative management after endoscopic resection of dysplastic polyps. *Gastroenterology.* 1999;117(6):1295-1300.

23. Friedman S, Odze RD, Farraye FA. Management of neoplastic polyps in inflammatory bowel disease. *Inflamm Bowel Dis.* 2003;9(4):260-266.

24. Farraye FA, Waye JD, Moscandrew M, Heeren TC, Odze RD. Variability in the diagnosis and management of adenoma-like and non-adenoma-like dysplasia-associated lesions or masses in inflammatory bowel disease: an Internet-based study. *Gastrointest Endosc.* 2007;66(3):519-529.

25. Hurlstone DP, Brown S. Techniques for targeting screening in ulcerative colitis. *Postgrad Med J.* 2007;83(981):451-460.

26. Thorlacius H, Toth E. Role of chromoendoscopy in colon cancer surveillance in inflammatory bowel disease. *Inflamm Bowel Dis.* 2007;13(7):911-917.

27. Hurlstone DP, Kiesslich R, Thomson M, Atkinson R, Cross SS. Confocal chromoscopic endomicroscopy is superior to chromoscopy alone for the detection and characterisation of intraepithelial neoplasia in chronic ulcerative colitis. *Gut.* 2008;57(2):196-204.

SHOULD I BE USING CHROMO-ENDOSCOPY IN MY SURVEILLANCE COLONOSCOPY IN INFLAMMATORY BOWEL DISEASE? HOW AND WHICH AGENT? WOULD NARROW BAND IMAGING BE AN ALTERNATIVE FOR THIS?

David T. Rubin, MD, FACG, AGAF

Current guidelines for cancer prevention in ulcerative colitis (UC) and Crohn's colitis involve performing screening and surveillance colonoscopies in order to detect precancerous dysplasia. The detection of precancerous dysplasia is necessary in order to stratify patients for follow-up and proctocolectomy. An accurate diagnosis of dysplasia in colitis requires a number of critical steps, with the first being adequate identification during colonoscopy. Traditionally, it was believed that, unlike sporadic colorectal cancer derived from raised polypoid lesions in non-inflammatory bowel disease (IBD) patients, dysplasia in IBD was "invisible" during endoscopy and could only be diagnosed by a trained pathologist. Therefore, surveillance guidelines recommended random biopsies throughout the colon in order to sample the mucosal surface area. This strategy was based on the fact that dysplasia often occurred in multiple locations simultaneously (synchronous lesions), so random biopsies could find it. The guidelines have suggested a minimum of 33 biopsies to achieve a statistically meaningful negative predictive value of an exam.[1]

The practical implementation of this approach, however, has been challenged by the fact that it is time-consuming and seems quite inaccurate. As a result, it is not surprising to see that most gastroenterologists do not follow the guidelines,[2] and, in practice, pathologists may not be reviewing all of the biopsies obtained. Better methods of dysplasia detection are clearly needed. One approach that has been described in recent years is the enhancement of optical colonoscopy techniques using chromoendoscopy, dye-sprayed either on the mucosa or on electronic filtering to alter the reflected light from the colon in order to identify dysplasia more accurately. These approaches, if effective, could provide a more targeted sampling of the mucosa, reduce the number of biopsies required, and, therefore, reduce the time needed for the exam, ultimately modifying the follow-up recommendations for dysplasia under the premise that if you can find it much more accurately, the worry about missed lesions that could progress or be associated with colorectal cancer would be reduced.

Dye-spraying chromoendoscopy is the more commonly described approach. Investigators have used either indigo carmine dye or methylene blue. Indigo carmine is not absorbed and, therefore, provides an enhancement of surface architecture, but not necessarily the more detailed cytoplasm uptake and imaging compared to methylene blue, which is readily absorbed into the epithelial cells. There are reports that the methylene blue may induce inflammation, so some investigators and early adopting clinicians have preferred indigo carmine. The standard approach is to first perform colonoscopy to the cecum. Then, in an adequately cleaned colon, the dye is sprayed in segments throughout the bowel. In order to perform the most successful examination, some experienced investigators recommend a bowel relaxant (like glucagon) to prevent motion artifact.[3] During careful withdrawal of the scope, subtle raised lesions and architecturally distorted mucosa are identified for targeted biopsies. Using this approach with the additional benefit of confocal endomicroscopy, in 2007, Kiesslich and colleagues were able to clearly and accurately identify the presence of dysplasia in vivo.[4] Their examination with magnification and chromoendoscopy only took 11 minutes longer than standard colonoscopy, and it identified significantly more dysplasia than standard optical colonoscopy. Additional studies with chromoendoscopy demonstrate similar increased yields (Table 15-1).

Narrow band imaging is performed using electronic filtering of the red wavelengths of light and, in essence, is similar to indigo carmine dye-spraying in its general ability to enhance surface architecture, but it is an attractive option given its simplicity (just a switch on the image processor). However, small preliminary studies have not demonstrated a clear benefit of this approach (Figures 15-1, 15-2, and 15-3).[5]

If chromoendoscopy with dyes or narrow band imaging is clearly more successful at finding dysplasia than optical white light colonoscopy, why is it not yet a standard of care? There are a few reasons for this, including an uncertain learning curve for clinicians in practice, unclear long-term outcomes from this approach, and concerns about how much time and money it requires. In addition, two retrospective studies have demonstrated that dysplasia and cancer in chronic UC are visible with our existing white light optical colonoscopy technology.[6,7]

Therefore, at the current time, chromoendoscopy in colitis surveillance is not my standard practice. Although there remains a compelling need for more accurate detection and prevention methods, we still must perform scheduled surveillance examinations and targeted (as well as random) biopsies, all reviewed by an experienced pathologist.

Table 15-1

Chromoendoscopy for Dysplasia in Ulcerative Colitis

Author (Year)	Institution	# of UC Patients	Type of Imaging	Results	
				# of dysplastic lesions (chromo versus conventional)	Sensitivity / Specificity
Kiesslich (2003)	University of Mainz, Germany	263	Methylene blue	42 (32 versus 10)	93% sens. 93% spec.
Rutter (2004)	St. Mark's Hospital, Harrow, UK	100	Indigo carmine	7 (7 versus 0)	Not given
Hurlstone (2005)	The Royal Hallamshire Hospital, Sheffield, UK	350	Indigo carmine and magnification	93 (69 versus 24)	93% sens. 88% spec.
Kiesslich (2007)	University of Mainz, Germany	161	Confocal endomicroscopy	23 (19 versus 4)	94.7% sens. 98.3% spec. 97.8% accuracy
Dekker (2007)	Academic Medical Center, Amsterdam, Netherlands	42	Narrow band imaging	15 (8 versus 7)	Not given

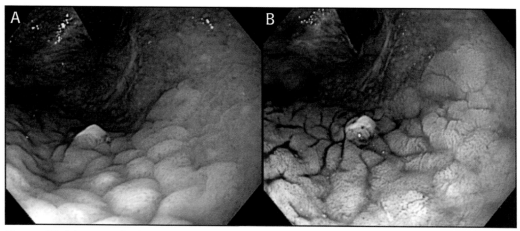

Figure 15-1. Low-grade dysplastic lesion in the rectum on retroflexion with optical colonoscopy (A), and after indigo carmine dye spraying (B).

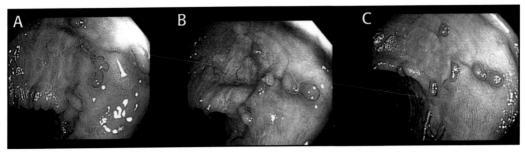

Figure 15-2. Ulcerative colitis patient with inflammatory polyps and melanosis coli on optical colonoscopy (A), with narrow band imaging (B), and after indigo carmine dye spray (C).

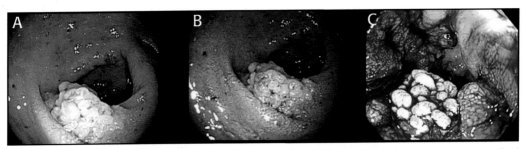

Figure 15-3. Long-standing ulcerative colitis with a dysplasia-associated mass lesion identified with white light (A), narrow band imaging (B), and methylene blue (C).

References

1. Kornbluth A, Sachar DB. Ulcerative colitis practice guidelines in adults (update): American College of Gastroenterology, Practice Parameters Committee. *Am J Gastroenterol.* 2004;99(7):1371-1385.
2. Bernstein CN WW, Levine DS, Shanahan F. Physicians' perceptions of dysplasia and approaches to surveillance colonoscopy in ulcerative colitis. *Am J Gastroenterol.* 1995;90(12):2106-2114.
3. Kiesslich R, Hoffman A, Neurath MF. Colonoscopy, tumors and inflammatory bowel disease—new diagnostic methods. *Endoscopy.* 2006;38(1):5-10.
4. Kiesslich R, Goetz M, Lammersdorf K, et al. Confocal endomicroscopy in dysplasia detection in chronic ulcerative colitis. *Gastroenterology.* 2007;132(3):874-882.
5. Dekker E, van den Broek FJ, Reitsma JB, et al. Narrow-band imaging compared with conventional colonoscopy for the detection of dysplasia in patients with longstanding ulcerative colitis. *Endoscopy.* 2007;39(3):216-221.
6. Rutter MD, Saunders BP, Wilkinson KH, Kamm MA, Williams CB, Forbes A. Most dysplasia in ulcerative colitis is visible at colonoscopy. *Gastrointest Endosc.* 2004;60(3):334-339.
7. Rubin DT, Rothe JA, Hetzel JT, Cohen RD, Hanauer SB. Is dysplasia visible during colonoscopy in UC? *Gastrointest Endosc.* 2007;65(7):998-1004.

CAN WE FOLLOW FLAT LOW-GRADE DYSPLASIA? IS ANY DYSPLASIA REALLY FLAT OR JUST A SPECTRUM OF DEPTH AND SIZE?

Arun Swaminath, MD and Thomas A. Ullman, MD, FACG

Precisely when to recommend colectomy has remained a topic of concern since the institution of colonoscopic dysplasia surveillance in inflammatory bowel disease (IBD). Since patients with high-grade dysplasia (HGD) carry an approximately 50% chance of already harboring colorectal cancer, almost no one questions the wisdom of offering a colectomy to these patients. In addition, the complete endoscopic resection of polypoid dysplastic lesions has gained near-universal acceptance as an alternative to colectomy. Flat low-grade dysplasia (LGD), however, presents more of a challenge to both patients and clinicians.

There are several important questions that patients and clinicians should ask when faced with flat LGD:

1. How accurate is a pathologist's diagnosis of LGD?
2. Was it really "flat" (or occult) neoplasia that was detected, or was it a subtly raised lesion that was unapparent to the endoscopist?
3. What is the risk of already harboring a colorectal malignancy that was missed at the time of colonoscopy?
4. What is the risk of progression to cancer if the patient pursues a nonoperative course?

The interpretation of biopsy specimens in ulcerative colitis (UC) patients can pose a challenge, even to expert pathologists. In an effort to standardize the histopathologic findings, the Inflammatory Bowel Disease Study Group issued a consensus manuscript in 1983 that defined levels of dysplasia in the colitis-dysplasia-carcinoma sequence.[1] Current histopathologic interpretations are based on this seminal report. Despite this codification, rates of observer agreement (even among expert gastrointestinal [GI] pathologists) have been less than ideal (especially in the intermediate grades of dysplasia), and indefinite for dysplasia and its subcategories and LGD. In one study among experts, crude rates of agreement ranged from 42% to 65%.[2] Hence, it is imperative that the gastroenterologist confer with the pathologist in cases of dysplasia, and that the findings are confirmed by a second pathologist (preferably at an expert center) prior to clinical decision making.

The current practice of surveillance in UC involves random and targeted (for visible lesions) biopsies. It is worth noting that even with the recommended 4 quadrant biopsies every 10 cm, less than 1% of the colonic mucosa is sampled. In addition, chart review and questionnaire-based studies have suggested that few gastroenterologists obtain the 33 biopsies needed to detect the presence of dysplasia with 90% certainty, as demonstrated by Rubin and colleagues.[3]

"Flat LGD" has come to mean LGD that is found in non-targeted biopsies. Whether it is truly flat or manifests different superficial features than polypoid features remains an area of uncertainty. Recent reports from St. Mark's in the United Kingdom and the University of Chicago in the United States have demonstrated that more and more detected dysplasia is visible rather than occult, suggesting that with changing scope optics, less dysplasia is coming from non-targeted (sometimes called "random") biopsies. As the natural history of these 2 distinct forms of dysplasia (occult and polypoid) are different in the published literature, recommendations on how to proceed are also different. As with the management of sporadic polypoid dysplasia, an incomplete resection of dysplastic lesions is a set-up for the development of malignancy. With the advent of chromoendoscopic techniques, even less dysplasia will prove to be flat, and the impact of complete resection of dysplastic tissue will become the norm. (The management of polypoid dysplasia is reviewed in Question 14 on page 57.)

Another key point in the management of flat LGD is the concept of a "field effect" for dysplasia in colitis. When dysplasia is found, there is no guarantee that a malignancy won't arise from a different portion of the colon than where the LGD was found—the entire colorectum is simultaneously at risk. This concept has been supported by the reality of a greater number of synchronous cancers at colectomy for both Crohn's colitis and UC, relative to sporadic colorectal cancer and the initial discovery of dysplasia by Morson and Pang in which rectal dysplasia was noted in the rectum of patients with more proximal malignancies.[4] Also in support of the field effect is the finding by 3 separate authors that for patients with LGD who have undergone colectomy within 6 months of their finding, an astonishing 20% harbor a malignancy. Such a high rate of synchronous cancer simultaneously supports the concept of the field effect and the recommendation that patients with LGD should be urged to undergo colectomy.

For patients who have elected to pursue a non-operative course following the detection of flat LGD, the data are varied. While US-based centers have demonstrated rates of progression to more advanced neoplasia ranging from 30% to 50% at 5 years, and some with progression to node positive cancers without intervening HGD, others have demonstrated a much more benign prognosis. Differences in histopathologic interpretation, inclusion of patients whose dysplasia was discovered prior to the 1983 classification scheme of the IBD Study Group, and differences in study size constitute the most likely reasons for these differences. Nevertheless, the uncertain prognosis of patients with flat LGD followed in surveillance makes a non-operative course a risky endeavor.

While it is certainly possible that new techniques such as chromoendoscopy (in which dye sprays such as indigo carmine or methylene blue are sprayed on the involved colorectum to better define highlight surface abnormalities) show promise in the detection of dysplasia in colitis, there are no longitudinal data to determine whether these techniques, or other evolving techniques like narrow band imaging, result in fewer colectomies and fewer cancer deaths. There is a suggestion that previously occult lesions will now be visible with these newer technologies. Recent data suggest that targeted biopsies using dye spray has a higher yield of dysplastic findings than those found by random biopsy.[5,6] In the future, occult lesions (currently encountered as flat dysplasia found on non-targeted biopsies) may be redefined as those that evade detection, despite the use of these newer technologies.

When faced with a patient with a new diagnosis of flat LGD, we recommend the following:

1. Have an expert GI pathologist confirm the finding. When patients are referred to Mount Sinai, our practice is to have the actual biopsy slides reviewed by our own Pathology Department.

2. If confirmed, the published literature is reviewed with the patient. This must include the 20% likelihood of already harboring a malignancy, the 50% rate of progression to advanced neoplasia in the coming 5 years, and the finding that, despite continued surveillance, some patients have developed node-positive cancers without any intervening abnormalities.[7]

3. Hand the name and number of a colorectal surgeon to the patient for a consultation.

4. Give a concrete recommendation that surgery is the safest course of action vis-à-vis cancer prevention.

Should the patient continue to refuse colectomy, we recommend intensive colonoscopic surveillance with chromoendoscopy to be more certain that HGDs have not previously been missed within the colorectum. This is usually at an interval of every 3 months for the first year, followed by every 6 months indefinitely.

References

1. Riddell RH, Goldman H, Ransohoff DF, et al. Dysplasia in inflammatory bowel disease: standardized classification with provisional clinical applications. *Hum Pathol.* 1983;14(11):931-968.
2. Melville DM, Jass JR, Morson BC, et al. Observer study of the grading of dysplasia in ulcerative colitis: comparison with clinical outcome. *Hum Pathol.* 1989;20(10):1008-1014.
3. Rubin CE, Haggitt RC, Burmer GC, et al. DNA aneuploidy in colonic biopsies predicts future development of dysplasia in ulcerative colitis. *Gastroenterology.* 1992;103(5):1611-1620.
4. Morson BC, Pang LS. Rectal biopsy as an aid to cancer control in ulcerative colitis. *Gut.* 1967;8(5):423-434.
5. Kiesslich R, Fritsch J, Holtmann M, et al. Methylene blue-aided chromoendoscopy for the detection of intraepithelial neoplasia and colon cancer in ulcerative colitis. *Gastroenterology.* 2003;124(4):880-888.
6. Rutter MD, Saunders BP, Schofield G, Forbes A, Price AB, Talbot IC. Pancolonic indigo carmine dye spraying for the detection of dysplasia in ulcerative colitis. *Gut.* 2004;53(2):256-260.
7. Ullman T, Croog V, Harpaz N, Sachar D, Itzkowitz S. Progression of flat low-grade dysplasia to advanced neoplasia in patients with ulcerative colitis. *Gastroenterology.* 2003;125(5):1311-1319.

QUESTION

CAN MEDICATIONS LIKE FOLIC ACID, URSODEOXYCHOLIC ACID, OR 5-AMINOSALICYLIC ACIDS LOWER THE RISK OF COLORECTAL CANCER OR DYSPLASIA IN PATIENTS WITH INFLAMMATORY BOWEL DISEASE?

Bret A. Lashner, MD

Colorectal cancer is an important cause of mortality in inflammatory bowel disease (IBD) patients. Since therapy for colorectal cancer is not always effective, strategies for primary prevention, when effective, should strongly be considered. Primary prevention in IBD patients through chemoprevention with 5-aminosalicylic acid (5-ASA), folic acid, and ursodeoxycholic acid (UDCA) has been studied.

5-AMINOSALICYLIC ACID

There are many theoretical reasons why 5-ASA agents could be chemopreventive for cancer or dysplasia. Five-ASA is known to inactivate reactive oxygen species and increase apoptosis through NF-κB suppression. Also, 5-ASA decreases interleukin 2 (IL-2) production, a cytokine known to stimulate clonal proliferation of T cells and epithelial cells. Five-ASA can also activate the peroxixome proliferator-activator receptor (PPAR)-γ, which is known to have both anti-inflammatory and anti-proliferative effects. By being a cyclooxygenase inhibitor, 5-ASA can be as chemopreventive as other non-steroidal anti-inflammatory drugs.

Many epidemiologic studies have examined a possible chemo-preventive effect from 5-ASA, and only about half have shown a statistically significant effect. A meta-analysis of all of these studies demonstrated a significant chemopreventive effect from 5-ASA (odds ratio [OR] 0.51, 95% CI 0.29-0.92) for the development of cancer or dysplasia.[1] Five-ASA is very often recommended for the maintenance of remission in ulcerative colitis (UC) patients. The likely chemo-preventive effect can be used to reinforce to patients the need to adhere to long-term therapy.

FOLIC ACID

Folic acid is essential for the regeneration of methionine, which is needed for purine and pyrimidine synthesis. Folate deficiency is associated with DNA hypomethylation, aberrant DNA synthesis and repair, and decreased apoptosis. Of note, folate-sensitive fragile sites exist on genes important for carcinogenesis, like the p53 suppressor gene. UC patients are particularly prone to be folic acid-deficient due to intestinal losses, poor intake, and competitive inhibition of absorption from sulfasalazine.

One case-control study examining this association found that for each 10 mg/mL increase in red blood cell folic acid, the risk of UC patients developing cancer or dysplasia was decreased by 18% (OR 0.82, 95% CI 0.68-0.99).[2] A cohort study showed a dose-response effect with folic acid supplementation (relative risk [RR] 0.76 for 0.4 mg folic acid daily and 0.54 for 1 mg folic acid daily).[3] The evidence is not strong, but since folic acid is inexpensive, safe, and recommended for the prevention of atherosclerotic heart disease, it too should be recommended for long-term use in IBD patients, either as a 0.4 mg component of a multivitamin, or as a 1.0 mg supplement.

URSODEOXYCHOLIC ACID

The risk of cancer and dysplasia is increased at least 3-fold in UC patients with primary sclerosing cholangitis (PSC).[4] Interestingly, the excess of cancers mostly occur on the right side of the colon when carcinogenic secondary bile acids, like deoxycholic acid, are increased. Theoretically, treating PSC patients with a primary bile acid such as UDCA should decrease the concentration of secondary bile acids and decrease the cancer risk.

Two epidemiologic studies looking at a possible chemopreventive effect from UDCA in PSC patients with UC came to opposite conclusions. Strong evidence, though, came from a randomized clinical trial on 52 UC patients with PSC being considered for UDCA treatment for liver disease.[5] The investigators found that dysplasia was detected in only 10% of UDCA-treated patients compared to 35% of placebo-treated patients (RR 0.26, 95% CI 0.06-0.92).[5] Currently, most PSC patients are treated with UDCA for their liver disease. Adherence to medical therapy could be improved if a possible cancer chemopreventive effect is discussed (Table 17-1).

CONCLUSION

The evidence is compelling that cancer chemoprevention should be a part of the regimen of all patients with UC and patients with extensive (at least 30% of the colon involved) Crohn's colitis who also are at risk for developing colorectal cancer. Even though patients may be in remission with other agents, such as infliximab or azathioprine, the added benefit of cancer chemoprevention should be considered. While chemoprevention can diminish the risk of cancer or dysplasia, the risk of malignancy is not eliminated, and cancer surveillance colonoscopy still needs to be performed. Until the magnitude of the

---

Table 17-1
Clinical Recommendations for Chemoprevention of Colorectal Cancer in Inflammatory Bowel Disease

1. All UC patients and patients with extensive Crohn's colitis should be offered 5-ASA at a minimimum of 2 g daily and folic acid at a minimum of 0.4 mg daily.
2. IBD patients with PSC should be offered UDCA at 20 mg/kg daily.
3. Cancer surveillance recommendations should continue at current 1- to 3-year intervals as clinically indicated.

---

risk reduction with chemoprevention is confirmed, testing intervals for cancer surveillance should not be lengthened, even in patients who are adherent to chemoprevention regimens.

References

1. Velayos FS, Terdiman JP, Walsh JM. Effect of 5-aminosalicylate use on cancer and dysplasia risk: a systematic review and meta-analysis of observational studies. *Am J Gastroenterol.* 2005;100(3):1345-1353.
2. Lashner BA. Red blood cell folate is associated with the development of dysplasia and cancer in ulcerative colitis. *J Cancer Res Clin Oncol.* 1993;119(9):549-554.
3. Lashner BA, Provencher KS, Seidner DL, et al. The effect of folic acid on the risk for cancer or dysplasia in ulcerative colitis. *Gastroenterology.* 1997;112(1):29-32.
4. Shetty K, Rybicki L, Brzezinski A, Carey WD, Lashner BA. The risk for cancer or dysplasia in ulcerative colitis patients with primary sclerosing cholangitis. *Am J Gastroenterol.* 1999;94(6):1643-1649.
5. Pardi DS, Loftus EV, Kremers WK, et al. Ursodeoxycholic acid as a chemopreventive agent in patients with ulcerative colitis and primary sclerosing cholangitis. *Gastroenterology.* 2003;124(4):889-893.

QUESTION 18

WHICH OF MY INFLAMMATORY BOWEL DISEASE PATIENTS SHOULD I SCREEN FOR OSTEOPOROSIS? SHOULD I ALSO SCREEN FOR VITAMIN D DEFICIENCY?

Kleanthis Dendrinos, MD and
Francis A. Farraye, MD, MSc, FACG, FASGE

Patients with inflammatory bowel disease (IBD) are at increased risk of bone loss. Bone mineral density (BMD) in IBD is influenced by a host of factors, including disease duration, severity of disease, age of onset, cumulative dose, duration of corticosteroid use, age, gender, and menopausal status in women (Table 18-1). Dual-energy x-ray absorptiometry scanning (DEXA) has proven to be an effective, safe, and inexpensive tool to noninvasively diagnose osteoporosis, a major risk factor for fracture in these patients. The American College of Gastroenterology (ACG) and American Gastroenterology Association (AGA) have both recently issued guidelines regarding the diagnosis of osteoporosis in patients with IBD.[1,2] These guidelines were evidence-based, with recommendations extrapolated in part from data in the postmenopausal osteoporosis literature, as well as from the rheumatology literature with regard to steroid-induced osteoporosis.

The 2003 guidelines recommended the selective screening of IBD patients with DEXA scanning if they have the following risk factors: postmenopausal women, ongoing steroid use, cumulative prior use of steroids greater than 3 months, a history of low trauma fractures, and an age over 60.

In 2006, Kornbluth and colleagues examined the utility of the guidelines in identifying the yield of bone loss.[3] They examined 100 consecutive outpatient IBD subjects over the age of 20 who underwent DEXA screening. The majority of the patients (90%) met the criteria for screening based on cumulative steroid use of greater than 3 months. Univariate analysis demonstrated that female gender, postmenopausal status, and low BMI were independent predictors of osteoporosis. Overall, they found that 44% of the patients had osteopenia, and 12% had osteoporosis. The results of DEXA screening changed manage-

---

Table 18-1

Risks Factors for Osteoporosis/Osteopenia in Inflammatory Bowel Disease Patients

- Postmenopausal women
- Ongoing steroid use
- Cumulative prior use of steroids greater than 3 months
- History of low trauma fractures
- Age over 60

---

ment in 66% of the patients screened. The most common therapy instituted was the initiation of calcium (1,500 mg/day) and vitamin D (600 IU/day) supplementation (66 patients), with 20 being started on risedronate for osteoporosis (12 patients) or osteopenia with ongoing steroid use (8 patients).

Our own unpublished data from 36 consecutive outpatients with Crohn's disease (CD) who were screened with DEXA demonstrated evidence of bone loss in 19 patients (53%). Of these, 16 had BMD scores consistent with osteopenia, and 3 with osteoporosis.

While BMD is a known risk factor for bone fracture, recent series have suggested that BMD alone is not an accurate predictor of fracture risk in the IBD population.[4] Other factors related perhaps to disease activity through associated cytokine release may also play a role. Another factor that is commonly used to assess bone health is vitamin D status.

Vitamin D supplements are available in two forms: vitamin D3 (cholecalciferol), which is produced in the skin through sun exposure, and vitamin D2 (ergocalcigerol), which is produced by the irradiation of ergosterol from yeast. Vitamin D2 is the form most commonly found in over-the-counter and prescription vitamin D supplements. In the body, both forms of vitamin D are transported to the liver, where they are metabolized to 25(OH)D (25-hydroxyvitamin D), which is measured in the serum to determine a person's vitamin D status.[5]

There is no formal definition of vitamin D deficiency. However, most experts agree that a serum level of 25(OH)D below 20 ng/mL constitutes vitamin D deficiency. Based on studies that show abnormal levels of parathyroid hormone and altered intestinal calcium transport at 25(OH)D levels below 29 ng/mL, a 25(OH)D level of 30 ng/mL or greater is considered by most authorities to be ideal. Vitamin D toxicity occurs at serum levels of 25(OH)D of 220 ng/mL or higher.[6]

The importance of vitamin D in the maintenance of healthy bone status is well known. However, it is increasingly being linked to other conditions as well. Adequate vitamin D levels are associated with a decrease in the rates of certain cancers.[7] The role of vitamin D in autoimmune diseases is also being elucidated. Based on epidemiologic studies and in animal models of IBD, there is evidence for a role of vitamin D in the regulation of the immune system of the gut.[8]

It is known that the prevalence of vitamin D deficiency is higher in IBD patients than in the general population. There is a 45% prevalence rate in ulcerative colitis (UC), and the

Table 18-2

Treatment of Vitamin D Deficiency in Patients With IBD

Cause of Deficiency	Preventive and Maintenance Measures to Avoid Deficiency	Treatment of Deficiency
Malabsorption syndromes (malabsorption of vitamin D, inadequate sun exposure, or supplementation)	Adequate exposure to sun or ultraviolet radiation; 50,000 IU of vitamin D2 every day, every other day, or every week; up to 10,000 IU of vitamin D3/day is safe for 5 months; maintenance dose is 50,000 IU of vitamin D2 every week*	UVB irradiation (tanning bed or portable UVB device (eg, portable Sperti lamp); 50,000 IU of vitamin D2 every day or every other day*

Adapted from Holick M.[9]

* The goal is to achieve concentrations of 25-hydroxyvitamin D at about 30 to 60 ng/mL. Physicians should use these guidelines in combination with their clinical judgment according to the circumstances.

prevalence rate for CD ranges from 22% to 77% in various studies.[10-12] Our own unpublished data examining vitamin D status in consecutive outpatient CD patients found a rate of vitamin D deficiency of 48% (14/29).

Several reasons for the increased rate of hypovitaminosis D in IBD have been proposed. These include decreased sun exposure, dietary restrictions, decreased absorption capacity, and increased GI loss.[13] Currently, there are no guidelines for the evaluation of vitamin D deficiency in patients with IBD. Furthermore, there are no consensus guidelines for the treatment of vitamin D deficiency in patients with IBD once the condition is discovered.

The Institute of Medicine currently recommends that children and adults up to the age of 50 have a daily dose of 200 IU/day of vitamin D. For those age 50 to 70 years, 400 IU/day is recommended, and a dose of 600 IU/day is recommended for those 70 years or older.[14] However, in those without adequate exposure to sunlight, most experts recommend a daily dose of 800 to 1000 IU of vitamin D to maintain adequate stores.[15]

The usual strategy for treating adults with vitamin D deficiency at our institution is to give 50,000 IU by mouth once weekly for 8 weeks, followed by 50,000 IU every 2 to 4 weeks for maintenance.[16]

As one of the possible reasons for the increased rate of vitamin D deficiency in CD may be diminished intestinal absorption capacity, alternate strategies for vitamin D supplementation for patients with evidence of malabsorption may be required (Table 18-2). To treat vitamin D deficiency in these patients, we give 50,000 IU of vitamin D2 every day or every other day for 3 weeks.[17] There have been several studies to support the safety of higher doses of vitamin D.[9] In cases that don't respond to oral supplementation, ultraviolet B (UVB) irradiation by means of a tanning bed may be necessary.[18] In these cases, we prescribe the patient spend 30% to 50% of the recommended time for tanning in the bed with sunscreen applied to the face.[19,20]

References

1. American Gastroenterology Association medical position statement: guidelines on osteoporosis in gastrointestinal disease. *Gastroenterology.* 2003;124(3):791-794.
2. Bernstein CN, Katz S. Guidelines for osteoporosis and inflammatory bowel disease: a guide to diagnosis and management for the gastroenterologist (monograph). *The American College of Gastroenterology.* 2003.
3. Kornbluth A, Hayes M, Feldman S, et al. Do guidelines matter? Implementation of ACG and AGA osteoporosis screening guidelines in IBD patients who meet the guidelines' criteria. *Am J Gastroenterol.* 2006;101(7):1546-1550.
4. Stockbrugger RW, Schoon EJ, Collani S, et al. Discordance between the degree of osteopenia and the prevalence of spontaneous vertebral fractures in Crohn's disease. *Aliment Pharmacol Ther.* 2002;16(8):1519-1527.
5. Holick MF, Garabedian M. Vitamin D: photobiology, metabolism, mechanism of action, and clinical applications. In: Favus MJ, ed. *Primer on the Metabolic Bone Diseases and Disorders of Mineral Metabolism.* 6th ed. Washington, DC: American Society for Bone and Mineral Research; 2006:129-137.
6. Holick MF. High prevalence of vitamin D inadequacy and implications for health. *Mayo Clin Proc.* 2006;81(3):353-373.
7. Feskanich D, Ma J, Fuchs CS, et al. Plasma vitamin D metabolites and risk of colorectal cancer in women. *Cancer Epidemiol Biomarkers Prev.* 2004;13(9):1502-1508.
8. Cantorna MT, Zhu Y, Froicu M, Wittke A. Vitamin D status, 1,25 dihydroxy vitamin D3, and the immune system. *Am J Clin Nutr.* 2004;80(suppl 6):1717S-1720S.
9. Holick MF. Vitamin D deficiency. *N Engl J Med.* 2007;357(3):266-281.
10. Siffledeen JS, Siminoski K, Steinhart H, et al. The frequency of vitamin D deficiency in adults with Crohn's disease. *Can J Gastroenterol.* 2003;17(8):473-478.
11. Tajika M, Matsuura A, Nakamura T, et al. Risk factors for vitamin D deficiency in patients with Crohn's disease. *J Gastroenterol.* 2004;39(8):527-533.
12. Silvennoinen J. Relationships between vitamin D, parathyroid hormone and bone mineral density in inflammatory bowel disease. *J Intern Med.* 1996;239(2):131-137.
13. Pappa HM, Grand RJ, Gordon CM. Report on the Vitamin D status of adult and pediatric patients with inflammatory bowel disease and its significance for bone health and disease. *Inflamm Bowel Dis.* 2006;12(12):1162-1174.
14. Standing Committee on the Scientific Evaluation of Dietary Reference Intakes Food and Nutrition Board, Institute of Medicine. Vitamin D. In: *Dietary Reference Intakes for Calcium, Phosphorus, Magnesium, Vitamin D, and Fluoride.* Washington, DC: National Academy Press; 1999:250-287.
15. Glerup H, Mikkelsen K, Poulsen L, et al. Commonly recommended daily intake of vitamin D is not sufficient if sunlight exposure is limited. *J Intern Med.* 2000;247(2):260-268.
16. Bouillon R. Vitamin D: from photosynthesis, metabolism, and action to clinical applications. In: DeGroot LJ, Jameson JL, eds. *Endocrinology.* Philadelphia, PA: W.B. Saunders; 2001:1009-1028.
17. Vieth R. Why the optimal requirement for vitamin D3 is probably much higher than what is officially recommended for adults. *J Steroid Biochem Mol Biol.* 2004;89-90(1-5):575-579.
18. Chel VGM, Ooms ME, Popp-Snijders C, et al. Ultraviolet irradiation corrects vitamin D deficiency and suppresses secondary hyperparathyroidism in the elderly. *J Bone Miner Res.* 1998;13(8):1238-1242.
19. Tangpricha V, Turner A, Spina C, Decastro S, Chen T, Holick MF. Tanning is associated with optimal vitamin D status (serum 25-hydroxyvitamin D concentration) and higher bone mineral density. *Am J Clin Nutr.* 2004;80(6):1645-1649.
20. Koutkia P, Lu Z, Chen TC, Holick MF. Treatment of vitamin D deficiency due to Crohn's disease with tanning bed ultraviolet B radiation. *Gastroenterology.* 2001;121(6):1485-1488.

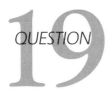
HOW DO YOU SCREEN AND SURVEY FOR DYSPLASIA IN CROHN'S PATIENTS? CAN YOU PERFORM SEGMENTAL RESECTION IN CROHN'S PATIENTS WITH DYSPLASIA?

Sonia Friedman, MD

Population- and hospital-based studies that span at least 35 years support an increased risk of colon cancer in patients with Crohn's disease (CD). Many of these papers, however, do not separate out the patients who are specifically at risk (those with extensive Crohn's colitis). One cannot compare the risk for colorectal cancer in CD with that of ulcerative colitis (UC) unless patients with equal extent and duration of disease are studied. Patients with only ileal disease or gastroduodenal disease have never been shown to have an increased risk of colorectal cancer. In studies that looked specifically at the risk of colorectal cancer in patients with Crohn's colitis, the standardized incidence ratio or the relative risk (RR), depending upon the study, is anywhere from 0.8 to 23.8.[1,2] In the only published surveillance program of 259 patients with Crohn's colitis,[3] there was a 22% chance of developing any low-grade dysplasia (LGD), high-grade dysplasia (HGD), or cancer by the fourth surveillance colonoscopy. Ninety percent of the patients in this study had extensive colitis, but all had more than a third of the colon involved. A recent study that followed the same group of patients for another 7 years reported a 25% chance of developing LGD, HGD, or cancer by the 10th surveillance exam, and a 7% chance of developing flat HGD or cancer by the 10th surveillance exam (Figure 19-1). There were 14 cancers found in this study—three on the screening exam and 11 on the surveillance exam or at surgery.[4] This is significantly more than is reported in the SEER (Surveillance, Epidemiology and End Results) registry as the number of cases of colorectal cancer that are expected in the general population (1.13).[5]

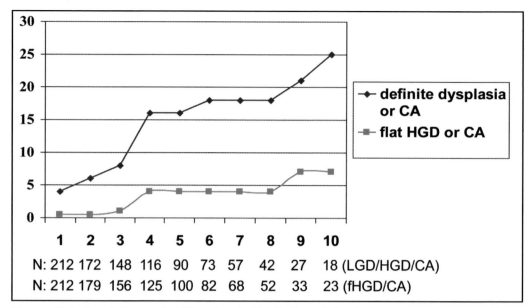

Figure 19-1. Cumulative probability of an initial finding of dysplasia or cancer on surveillance exams. CA = cancer. This figure was published in *Clin Gastroenterol Hepatol*. Friedman S, Rubin D, Bodian C, Harpaz N, Present DH. Screening and surveillance and surveillance colonoscopy in chronic colitis: results of a surveillance program spanning 25 years. 953-954. Copyright Elsevier (2008).

Given the increased incidence of colorectal cancer in Crohn's colitis, we do need to perform colonoscopic surveillance in these patients. I recommend an initial screening colonoscopy at 8 years after onset of symptoms in patients with at least one-third of the colon macroscopically or microscopically involved. Those patients at a higher risk for cancer have a large extent of disease (pancolitis), longer duration of disease, colonic strictures that are impassable with a pediatric colonoscope, and surgically bypassed segments of the colon. Other factors that further increase the risk of colorectal cancer are a personal history of primary sclerosing cholangitis, a family history of colon cancer, and a young age of disease onset. At screening colonoscopy, 4 quadrant biopsies should be performed every 10 cm, and biopsies should also be taken from strictures, suspicious lesions, and masses. All polypoid dysplastic lesions deemed "adenoma-like" can be totally removed. The bases of all polyps should be biopsied extensively, as well as the areas of mucosa surrounding each polyp. If endoscopy and pathology are negative, the exam should be repeated in 2 years.

If dysplasia is found, management is controversial. There is little hard data on the management of dysplasia and cancer in Crohn's colitis, and new imaging techniques such as dye spray, magnification, and high definition colonoscopy are unstudied in CD. For unifocal flat LGD in Crohn's colitis, the management is even more difficult than in UC. Many patients with Crohn's colitis have extensive ileal disease, and surgery would involve an extensive ileal resection, as well as a total proctocolectomy and standard Brooke ileostomy. This might predispose a patient to short bowel syndrome or, at the very least, trouble with fluid balance. Since doctors and patients alike are reluctant to choose such an extensive surgery, frequent surveillance is often more palatable. An alternative management would be to do another colonoscopy in 1 to 6 months with dye spray and a high-definition colonoscope. If recurrent or multifocal LGD is found, the patient will need surgery after confirming the results with a second pathologist. The usual surgeries performed for flat LGD are a total proctocolectomy and ileostomy, or a subtotal colectomy and ileo-rectal anastamosis. This latter surgery can be performed, of course, only if the dysplasia is not located in the rectum and as long as there is no active perianal fistulizing disease.

Flat HGD is a more serious lesion than flat LGD, and there is a higher likelihood of cancer elsewhere in the colon. If the location cannot be definitely ascertained, the patient will need an extensive resection. If the HGD occurs within a mass, and if there is no dysplasia elsewhere in the colon, a segmental resection can be considered. Before doing a segmental resection, however, it would be prudent to do another colonoscopy with dye spray and a high-definition colonoscope to make sure there is no other dysplasia. With this said, I would discuss with the patient that dysplasia usually occurs as a field effect, and where there is one lesion, there will likely be others in the future. For a mass containing cancer, the same principle would apply. In a patient with no microscopic or macroscopic CD elsewhere in the colon, it is probably safe to do a segmental resection. For a patient with pancolitis, it is less safe but reasonable to perform in a patient with extensive ileal disease or in a medically less fit patient who cannot tolerate major surgery. In one study, 3 patients with cancer had segmental resections even though they had pancolitis.[4] Five-year follow-up has been negative for recurrent dysplasia or cancer.

The management of polyps is exactly as in UC. Pedunculated polyps containing LGD, HGD, or cancer can be removed by snare cautery and followed by surveillance colonoscopies. Small sessile LGD polyps can be removed endoscopically, but consideration should be given to surgery in patients with large sessile polyps that are difficult to remove or smaller sessile polyps containing HGD or cancer.

For the field of management of dysplasia in chronic Crohn's colitis, the waters are almost uncharted. There is only a single study of a colonoscopic surveillance program spanning 25 years, but the results are by no means definitive. What makes Crohn's complicated is the extensive ileal disease and active perianal disease that these patients often have, making surgery less feasible. It is likely that with new technology, including chromoendoscopy, magnification endoscopy, and high-definition endoscopy, surgery will be performed less and less for LGD in CD. What is most important is that the same rules of surveillance apply for Crohn's as in UC—that patients with more than 8 years of disease duration and more than half of the colon involved undergo biennial colonoscopic surveillance.

References

1. Gyde SN, Prior P, Macartney JC, et al. Malignancy in Crohn's disease. *Gut*. 1980;21(12):1024-1029.
2. Jess T, Loftus E, Velayos F, et al. Risk of intestinal cancer in inflammatory bowel disease: a population-based study from Olmstead, Minnesota. *Gastroenterology*. 2006;130(4):1039-1046.
3. Friedman S, Rubin PH, Bodian C, Harpaz N, Present DH. Screening and surveillance colonoscopy on chronic Crohn's colitis. *Gastroenterology*. 2001;120(4):820-826.

4. Friedman S, Rubin PH, Bodian C, Harpaz N, Present DH. Screening and surveillance colonoscopy in chronic Crohn's colitis: results of a surveillance program spanning 25 years. *Clin Gastroenterol Hepatol.* 2008;6(9):993-998.

5. Ries LAG, Melbert D, Krapcho M, et al, eds. *SEER Cancer Statistics Review, 1975-2004.* Bethesda, MD: National Cancer Institute; 2007. Available at: http://seer.cancer.gov/csr/1975_2004/. Based on November 2006 SEER data submission, posted to the SEER web site, 2007.

WHAT SHOULD WE BE TELLING OUR PATIENTS AND THEIR PEDIATRICIANS ABOUT USING ANTI-TUMOR NECROSIS FACTOR ALPHA THERAPY DURING PREGNANCY?

Marla C. Dubinsky, MD

The benefits of infliximab have afforded more women of childbearing age the opportunity to successfully conceive and experience a normal pregnancy. Thus, we have entered into an era where more women who would have otherwise chosen to not get pregnant voluntarily or who could not due to uncontrolled disease are facing the scenario of how to manage the newborn that was exposed to infliximab throughout gestation. This remains a relatively novel clinical scenario for the gastroenterologists managing pregnant inflammatory bowel disease (IBD) patients, and something that the pediatricians now have to be aware of as well.

The infliximab product label in the United States states that "it is not known whether Remicade can cause fetal harm when administered to a pregnant woman." Based on the original animal studies, there was no evidence to suggest that engineered therapeutic antibodies administered to an expectant mother crossed the placenta to her offspring. However, the preclinical animal reproduction studies were not conducted with the actual infliximab antibody because infliximab does not cross-react with tumor necrosis factor alpha (TNF-α) in species other than human beings and chimpanzees. Thus, an analogous murine anti-TNF surrogate antibody was used by the manufacturer to conduct reproductive, developmental, and fertility toxicology studies in rodents. To move forward, studies need to be done using animal models in which infliximab would cross react with TNF-α. One such study was recently published using golimumab in pregnant macaques (a widely distributed genus of nonhuman primates).[1]

There is a transfer of immunoglobulin G (IgG) from maternal to fetal circulations before birth in primates, and the IgG1 subtype is maximally transported across the placenta during the third trimester, while peaking at term. These antibodies may take up to a year to be cleared by the offspring. Based on a case report that demonstrated evidence for transplacental transfer of maternally administered infliximab to the newborn, it would appear that infliximab is similarly cleared at a slower rate.[2] In this study, the newborn had detectable infliximab levels out to 6 months after birth. Of note, the drug level in the baby at 6 weeks of age was the same as the level measured in the mother at the same time who had received infliximab just 2 weeks prior to the serum acquisition, and who had also received an infusion 4 weeks before delivery. It was suggested that perhaps the infliximab was transferred in the breast milk. However, there were no detectable levels of the drug in the breast milk. Moreover, in humans, the amount of IgG1 secreted in breast milk is minimal. Despite persistence with breastfeeding, the infant's levels continued to decrease over the 6-month monitoring period. The conclusion from this study was that infliximab was actively transported across the placenta and not via the breast milk. Further research confirms that infliximab levels in the cord blood are reflective of the level in the newborn, suggesting further that infliximab does indeed cross the placenta in humans.[3]

Exposure in utero is one thing, but now we must also come to understand the implications of measurable infliximab in the serum of newborns and how this potentially impacts the maturing immune system. It remains unknown as to how long after placental exposure we should concern ourselves about the potential immunomodulatory effects on the newborn. TNF-α is known to be important for the developing immune system, and therefore, prolonged exposure to an antibody that neutralizes the biologic activity of TNF-α during the critical time period of immune system development raises potential concerns. In TNF-α knockout mice, there is evidence of poor formation of the secondary structures of lymphoid organs. This is important because the formation of germinal centers is a critical step in the humoral immune responses that depends on the cooperative effects of B and T cells. It is unknown whether this has the same implications in the developing human fetal humoral immune system. Thus, further knowledge is needed as to whether anti–TNF-α antibody exposure during the perinatal period and during the early months of immune system development could result in less obvious longer-term implications.

The newborn from the case report described above had a comprehensive immune evaluation at 6 months of age, and the results suggested age-appropriate immune development, including normal ability to mount appropriate immune response to routine childhood immunizations (Table 20-1). A follow-up study performed in a larger cohort of infants confirms the previously observed minimal effect of infliximab on the developing immune system. This is in keeping with the most recent data obtained from a primate study that used golimumab in macaques. This study showed that in utero and postnatal exposure to golimumab had no effect on T and B cell populations in blood and lymphoid tissues, and it did not impair the ability of the infants to mount an immune response to antigen challenge. Similar results applied to golimumab use during lactation. More human data is definitely needed to feel comfortable with the safety of perinatal anti–TNF-α exposure.

Table 20-1

Immune Studies Performed at Six Months of Age

- T & B lymphocyte subsets normal
- Total IgG, IgM, and IgA concentrations normal for age
- Normal in vitro lymphoproliferative responses to nonspecific mitogens
    Phytohemagglutinin
    Pokeweed mitogen
- Normal, protective levels of antibodies to protein and conjugated polysaccharide vaccines
    Hemophilus influenza type b (Hib)
    Streptococcus pneumoniae
    Tetanus

The lack of data in humans breeds the question of which vaccinations are safe to administer during the first 12 months of life. The killed vaccines such as hemophilus influenza type B, tetanus, diphtheria, pertussis, and hepatitis B are recommended to all infants, irrespective of exposures during pregnancy and lactation. The live vaccines, however, as is the case in all patients with IBD receiving immunosuppressive therapies, could present a problem for infants exposed in utero. The only live vaccine that is now recommended for infants below the age of 12 months is the rotavirus vaccine. Until we have more information as to the effects, or lack thereof, for anti–TNF-α exposure in utero and during lactation on the maturing immune system, administration of the rotavirus vaccine may not be prudent. That being said, the risk of not vaccinating and the actual risk of rotavirus to infants (eg, in the face of specific high risk factors such as socioeconomic status, attendance at daycare, and exposure to siblings) must also be taken into consideration. This needs to be discussed with the mother and pediatrician, and consulting an infectious disease physician may be considered. By 12 months of age, when the varicella vaccine and Measles, Mumps, and Rubella (MMR) vaccine are due, the infant should not still have the remnant effects of anti–TNF-α therapies. It is recommended that at 7 months of age, newborns exposed to anti–TNF-α in utero should minimally have confirmation of mounting a protective immune response to the killed vaccines. Titers of antibodies to tetanus toxoid and hemophilus influenza type B can be tested, and, if undetectable, the infant should receive a booster shot to be protected.

It has been suggested that, given infliximab is transported maximally during the last trimester, exposure should be minimized during this period, perhaps with the last infusion before delivery to be administered around 30 weeks of gestation. Obviously, that can be more difficult in patients receiving adalimumab, but some clinicians have suggested stopping 8 weeks before delivery, and then resuming either medication immediately postpartum if possible, but this must be evaluated on a case-by-case basis. Thus, limiting placental transfer will limit exposure to the fetus, which would lead to minimal effect on the developing immune system. Infliximab (not adalimumab) levels are measurable, so physicians should consider measuring infliximab levels within 2 months of delivery and following the levels until undetectable to feel more comfortable with exposing infants to live vaccines.

This is certainly an evolving field, and, as a result of improved management, an increasing number of patients are planning and carrying successful pregnancies. Therefore, a growing interest is being paid to the possible consequences of IBD and associated immunosuppressive therapies (anti–TNF-α, in particular) on the fetus and newborn infant.

References

1. Martin PL, Oneda S, Treacy G. Effects of an anti-TNF-alpha monoclonal antibody, administered throughout pregnancy and lactation, on the development of the macaque immune system. *Am J Reprod Immunol.* 2007;58(2):138-149.
2. Vasiliauskas EA, Church JA, Silverman N, Barry M, Targan SR, Dubinsky MC. Case report: evidence for transplacental transfer of maternally administered infliximab to the newborn. *Clin Gastroenterol Hepatol.* 2006;4(10):1255-1258.
3. Mahadevan U, Terdiman J, Church J, et al. Infliximab levels in infants born to women with inflammatory bowel disease. *Gastroenterol.* 2007;132:A-144.

WHAT ARE THE RISKS TO THE FETUS AND TO THE BABY REGARDING AZATHIOPRINE AND 6-MERCAPTOPURINE IN PREGNANCY AND NURSING?

Uma Mahadevan-Velayos, MD

When I discuss medical therapy during pregnancy and lactation with a woman with inflammatory bowel disease (IBD), I focus on the individual risks and benefits to that patient—is she in remission? for how long? what are her concomitant medications? etc. Globally, the current consensus in gastroenterology is that azathioprine and 6-mercaptopurine (6-MP) are low-risk for use during pregnancy, and are possibly compatible with breastfeeding as well. Six-MP and its pro-drug azathioprine are Food and Drug Administration (FDA) pregnancy category D agents. This means that positive evidence of fetal risk is available, but the benefits may outweigh the risk if life-threatening or serious disease exists. Providing up-to-date information to the patient prior to pregnancy is ideal so that appropriate adjustments can be made and the stress of the situation can be reduced for the parents and the treating physician. Also, one will not be in the situation of treating an acutely flaring pregnant woman who stopped her medications on her own when she found out she was pregnant! I discuss the information presented here and in Table 21-1 with my patients.

Animal studies, in which supratherapeutic doses are given intraperitoneally or intravenously (IV), have demonstrated teratogenicity with increased frequencies of cleft palate, open-eye, and skeletal anomalies seen in mice exposed to azathioprine, and cleft palate, skeletal anomalies, and urogenital anomalies seen in rats.[1] Transplacental and transamniotic transmission of azathioprine and its metabolites from the mother to the fetus can occur. However, in humans, the oral bioavailability of azathioprine (47%) and 6-MP (16%) is low, and the early fetal liver lacks the enzyme inosinate pyrophosphorylase needed to convert azathioprine to 6-MP.[1] Both of these features may protect the fetus from toxic drug exposure during the crucial period of organogenesis (first 8 weeks of gestation).

Table 21-1
Main Points

- Azathioprine and 6-MP are considered low-risk in pregnancy based on data in IBD, liver transplantation, and other autoimmune diseases.
- Recent data have been conflicting with respect to whether there may[2] or may not be[3] an increased risk of congenital anomalies.
- Continue azathioprine/6-MP if this is the sole agent maintaining remission.
- You can consider stopping azathioprine/6-MP if it is only being used to reduce immunogenicity to a biologic agent and the latter is the primary therapeutic agent.
- Azathioprine/6-MP may now be compatible with breastfeeding as serum levels of metabolites are not detected in the breastfeeding infant.

The largest evidence on safety comes from transplantation studies, where rates of anomalies ranged from 0 to 11.8%, and no evidence of recurrent patterns of congenital anomalies emerged. A population-based cohort study from Denmark[4] compared 11 women exposed to azathioprine or 6-MP with the general population (19,418 controls). The adjusted odds ratio (OR) for congenital malformations was 6.7 (95% CI, 1.4-32.4). However, when a single severely ill patient with autoimmune hepatitis and multiple other medications was removed from the cohort, the OR was 3.4 (95% CI, 0.4-27.3).

In IBD, multiple-case series have not noted an increase in congenital anomalies. Recently, however, a Danish nationwide cohort study by Norgard[2] found that women with Crohn's disease (CD) exposed to corticosteroids and azathioprine/6-MP were more likely to have a preterm birth (12.3% and 25%, respectively) compared to non-IBD controls (6.5%). Congenital anomalies were also more prevalent among azathioprine- and 6-MP–exposed cases compared to the reference group (15.4% versus 5.7%) with an OR of 2.9 (95% CI 0.9-8.9). Only 26 women were exposed to azathioprine/6-MP during conception versus 628 patients in the reference group. The largest study to date was by Goldstein, et al.[3] In this study, 189 women who called one of 7 teratogen information services for exposure to azathioprine in pregnancy were compared to 230 women who also called, but had no teratogenic drug exposure. The rate of major malformations was the same between the two groups: azathioprine (3.5%) versus controls (3.0%) (p = .775; OR 1.17; CI: 0.37, 3.69).

With respect to breastfeeding, given the potential for severe toxicity in the breastfeeding infant, breastfeeding is not recommended by the American Academy of Pediatrics (AAP). However, recent small studies in IBD suggest that the overall exposure to the infant is low. In one study of 4 women breastfeeding on azathioprine, 2 women had multiple breast milk samples that did not have detectable levels of drug by high-performance liquid chromatography. Two other studies measured metabolite levels in the breastfeeding infant. One reported 4 infants with undetectable metabolite levels, despite mothers whose levels were in the therapeutic range.[5] Sau collected 31 samples from 10 breastfeeding women on azathioprine and 6-MP.[6] Only 2 samples had low levels of 6-MP in breast milk (1.2 and 7.6 ng/mL in one patient versus a serum level of 50 ng/mL). There was no detectable 6-thioguanine nucleotides (6-TGN) or 6-methylmercaptopurine (6-MMP) levels in the 10 infants, nor were there signs of hematologic or clinical immunosuppression. Overall, these three studies suggest that the transfer of the drug to the breastfeeding infant is minimal. The risks and benefits of breastfeeding must be considered carefully. However, there does not appear to be an absolute contraindication to breastfeeding.

A patient who is on azathioprine or 6-MP is on it because at one time she had moderate to severe disease. If she stops her medication, she has a good chance of having her disease recur during the course of the pregnancy. As one of our primary goals remains the health of the mother, I do encourage women on azathioprine/6-MP to continue this agent during pregnancy given the risk profile noted above. One exception is for the patient on azathioprine/6-MP to reduce the immunogenicity of her biologic therapy. In this situation, in the completely stable patient, I will offer to stop the azathioprine/6-MP. Another exception is that I do not start azathioprine/6-MP for the first time during pregnancy. As we cannot predict who will have pancreatitis, bone marrow suppression, and other severe side effects, the time to try it out is not during pregnancy! It is always a risk-to-benefit evaluation, and in these 2 cases, the risks may outweigh the benefit.

Another problem is that certain obstetricians refuse to take care of patients on this medication. I recommend that all women with IBD be followed as high-risk pregnancies given their increased risks of preterm birth, low birth weight, and complications of labor, regardless of medications used and disease activity.[7] Most maternal-fetal medicine (high-risk obstetric) specialists are comfortable following the patient on azathioprine/6-MP as they are aware of the global issues with the disease. Breastfeeding is a different issue. The lack of data on the transfer in breast milk is limited, and many mothers do not feel comfortable with this situation. I present the data stated above to the mothers, and they decide whether they want to breastfeed. I do not recommend stopping the azathioprine to breastfeed, as many of my patients have had severe flares in this setting.

The decision is ultimately the mother's, and given the appropriate education, most of them choose to continue the medication if it is their sole means of maintaining remission. In my practice, most choose not to breastfeed.

References

1. Polifka JE, Friedman JM. Teratogen update: azathioprine and 6-mercaptopurine. *Teratology*. 2002;65(5):240-261.
2. Norgard B, Pedersen L, Christensen LA, Sorensen HT. Therapeutic drug use in women with Crohn's disease and birth outcomes: a Danish nationwide cohort study. *Am J Gastroenterol*. 2007;102(7):1406-1413.
3. Goldstein LH, Dolinsky G, Greenberg R, et al. Pregnancy outcome of women exposed to azathioprine during pregnancy. *Birth Defects Res A Clin Mol Teratol*. 2007;79(10):696-701.
4. Norgard B, Pedersen L, Fonager K, Rasmussen SN, Sorensen HT. Azathioprine, mercaptopurine and birth outcome: a population-based cohort study. *Aliment Pharmacol Ther*. 2003;17(6):827-834.
5. Gardiner SJ, Gearry RB, Roberts RL, Zhang M, Barclay ML, Begg EJ. Exposure to thiopurine drugs through breast milk is low based on metabolite concentrations in mother-infant pairs. *Br J Clin Pharmacol*. 2006;62(4):453-456.
6. Sau A, Clarke S, Bass J, Kaiser A, Marinaki A, Nelson-Piercy C. Azathioprine and breastfeeding: is it safe? *Bjog*. 2007;114(4):498-501.
7. Mahadevan U, Sandborn WJ, Li DK, Hakimian S, Kane S, Corley DA. Pregnancy outcomes in women with inflammatory bowel disease: a large community-based study from Northern California. *Gastroenterology*. 2007;133(4):1106-1112.

MY 25-YEAR-OLD PATIENT WITH CROHN'S DISEASE ON AZATHIOPRINE WAS RECENTLY DIAGNOSED WITH HPV. IS IT SAFE TO CONTINUE THE AZATHIOPRINE?

Sunanda Kane, MD, MSPH, FACG, FACP, AGAF

Human papillomavirus (HPV) infection can manifest in a variety of different clinical conditions. Some are benign and others can be quite serious.[1]

First, let us take the scenario where a patient has small, painless lesions on his hands.[2] On examination, they are pearly white, can be single or multiple, and occur on the dorsal aspect of the hand and lateral parts of the digits. These are classic warts and can be treated with over-the-counter medications or liquid nitrogen in a physician's office. If they are recurrent, grow larger, or cause pain, they should be evaluated by a dermatologist. Warts are a result of HPV infection and are more unsightly than dangerous. Since the majority of the lesions can easily be cauterized and eradicated, the benefits of the azathioprine therapy may considerably outweigh the risks in this case.

Now let's assume that this patient is a woman and that the HPV was found on cervical cytology. When a woman is diagnosed with an HPV infection, it is important to know whether this is associated with any dysplasia or cellular atypia. If there is dysplasia, then minimizing immune suppression may become very important. The HPV should be serotyped, as serotypes 16 and 18 are clearly associated with the development of cancer and require closer monitoring. If the HPV infection is found without dysplasia, then cessation may not be mandated. Other risk factors for dysplasia include sexual promiscuity, cigarette smoking, and the use of oral contraceptives. Patients with Crohn's disease (CD) tend to smoke more than the normal population. Thus, smoking cessation should be part of a treatment plan for both the cervical dysplasia as well as the CD. Oral contraceptive use has been associated with more aggressive cervical lesions and should also be stopped.

There are recent data to suggest that women with inflammatory bowel disease (IBD) have a higher risk of abnormal cervical cytology as compared to the healthy population. This relationship does not include cervical cancer, however, most likely because lesions are found early and appropriate intervention takes place. This increased risk has been associated specifically with immunomodulator use and not with biologics. This patient is 25, and according to the most recently published guidelines from the American College of Obstetrics and Gynecology, she is an appropriate candidate for Gardasil (Merck & Co., Inc., Whitehouse, NJ) treatment regardless of whether she is HPV positive.[3] The immuno-suppression does not need to be stopped unless she has a history of an advanced cervical lesion. Unlike for warts, cervical dysplasia can be more serious, and the indication for azathioprine needs to be reassessed. Minimizing immunosuppression will be important in preventing progression of the cervical lesion or its recurrence. If there are alternatives, they certainly should be used while the HPV is being eradicated. Alternatives to consider would be biologic therapy or surgery. It is unclear if methotrexate (MTX) carries the same risk for viral replication as the anti-metabolites. If no other reasonable options exist, then I would decrease the dose to the lowest amount possible. In this scenario, if the patient has required cervical cautery and recurrence has not been ruled out, perhaps even surgery (if the disease is limited) should be considered to allow for eradication over a few months' time.

The third scenario to consider is that of HPV infection in the setting of anal warts. The potential for cancer in this setting is also increased. Again, if the lesions are associated with dysplasia, then immunosuppression should be minimized while still maintaining remission.[4] While there is an increased risk for squamous cell cancer in the anal canal with HPV, there has been no data to suggest this risk is higher in the IBD patient popula-tion. However, these are relatively old studies, and no mention of chronic immunosup-pression is made. Cancer can occur in the epithelium of perianal fistulous tracts, but not associated with HPV infection or chronic immunosuppression use. There is a recent report of dysplasia found in the rectum of a patient with long standing ulcerative colitis (UC) treated with 6-mercaptopurine (6-MP) that was found to be HPV-16 positive. Clearly, if lesions within the mucosa or epithelium are identified that are associated with dyspla-sia and HPV infection, then trying to minimize immunosuppression is important, and cessation of azathioprine is a serious consideration.

References

1. Nindl I, Gottschling M, Stockfleth E. Human papillomaviruses and non-melanoma skin cancer: basic virology and clinical manifestations. *Dis Markers*. 2007;23(4):247-259.
2, Kane SV, Khatibi B, Reddy D. Higher incidence of abnormal pap smears in women with inflammatory bowel disease. *Am J Gastroenterol*. 2008;103(3):631-636.
3. Wright TC, Massad LS, Dunton CJ, et al. 2006 consensus guidelines for the management of women with abnormal cervical cancer screening tests. *Am J Obstet Gynecol*. 2007;197(4):346-355.
4. Frisch M, Gimelius B, van den Brule AJ, et al. Benign anal lesions, inflammatory bowel disease and risk for high-risk human papillomavirus-positive and -negative anal carcinoma. *Br J Cancer*. 1998;78(11):1534-1538.

WHAT IS THE ROLE OF COMPUTED TOMOGRAPHIC ENTEROGRAPHY IN THE DIAGNOSIS AND MANAGEMENT OF INFLAMMATORY BOWEL DISEASE? HAS IT REPLACED BARIUM RADIOGRAPHY?

Edward V. Loftus, Jr., MD

Inflammatory bowel disease (IBD) remains a collection of idiopathic syndromes that are diagnosed by the clinician. There is no one single test that is pathognomonic for IBD, and the clinician must integrate the results of multiple streams of information to produce a diagnosis. In addition to the history and physical examination, the diagnosis typically has rested on the results of colonoscopy and/or ileoscopy with biopsy and barium examination of the small bowel, also known as small bowel follow-through (SBFT). At many centers, however, SBFT has been largely replaced by an examination known as computed tomography enterography (CTE). The hallmarks of this procedure include oral ingestion of a large volume (ie, at least 1400 mL) of a neutral oral contrast agent to optimize small bowel distension and provide a contrast between the lumen and the wall of the small intestine, intravenous (IV) administration of iodinated contrast, and acquisition of thin slices of images throughout the abdomen and pelvis.[1] In Crohn's disease (CD), the typical findings on CTE include mural hyperenhancement, mural stratification, increased mural thickness or asymmetry, fibrofatty proliferation, increased mesenteric fat density, and the "comb sign" (ie, engorged vasa recta) (Figure 23-1).

Some studies suggest an increased sensitivity of CTE for active small bowel inflammation relative to SBFT, and this is not surprising considering that CD is a transmural, not merely mucosal, process.[2] The aforementioned radiographic findings track well with other measures of CD activity such as ileal erosions on endoscopy or elevated serum C-reactive protein (CRP) concentrations.[3,4] One prospective blinded study of diagnostic

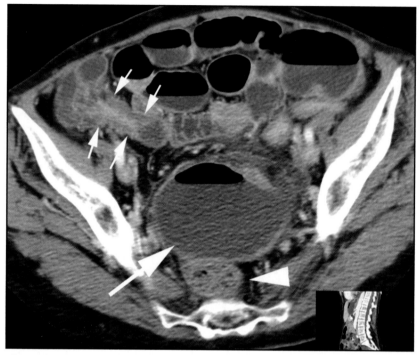

Figure 23-1. CTE of the abdomen and pelvis in a patient with Crohn's disease, which reveals mural thickening, hyperenhancement, and luminal narrowing of the terminal ileum (small arrows), and marked proximal small bowel dilation (large arrow) indicating significant partial small bowel obstruction. Arrowhead indicates rectum. Image courtesy of JG Fletcher, MD.

modalities in patients with known or suspected CD suggested that CTE was more sensitive in detecting active small bowel CD than ileoscopy or SBFT, although these differences were not statistically significant.[5] Furthermore, CTE was found to be more specific than capsule endoscopy. CTE also has the advantage of detecting occult small bowel strictures that might have resulted in the impaction of an endoscopy capsule. One retrospective study suggested that the prevalence of penetrating disease in 357 consecutive patients with known CD who underwent CTE was over 20%, and that the penetrating complication was a new finding in over half of these.[6] Moreover, almost 20% of these patients had evidence of extraintestinal manifestations or complications of IBD, and approximately two-thirds of these findings were new.

CTE is not for every patient with known or suspected CD. The lack of adequate bowel distension and the lack of IV contrast both severely limit CTE's utility, so patients who cannot ingest the relatively large volume of oral contrast or who cannot receive iodinated IV contrast (renal insufficiency, severe contrast dye allergy) should undergo alternative imaging. Some have raised concerns about the cost of CTE relative to SBFT. While it is true that CTE is significantly more expensive than SBFT, many believe that the increased amount of information it gleans and the resultant changes in patient management are well worth the increased cost. Indeed, one study suggested that CTE changed the ordering clinicians' perception of corticosteroid benefit in over half of patients with CD.[7] Nevertheless, additional prospective studies that better quantify the added value of CTE and how it changes patient management are required. A second concern that has been raised about CTE has been the increased exposure of the patient to ionizing radiation. The effective dose of radiation received by the patient during CTE is estimated to be 3 to 4 times higher than that received during SBFT. Indeed, we found in a population-based cohort that, although the average cumulative dose of ionizing radiation from diagnostic procedures was not much higher than what one would expect from background radiation, the doses received by the top quartile of patients was significantly higher, and much of this increase could be explained by the increasing use of CT.[8] Hopefully, this issue will become less clinically relevant with the refinement of CT dose-reduction techniques, particularly in patients requiring serial imaging. Our radiologists have already been able to reduce the effective dose of radiation by approximately 30%, and it is expected that further dose reductions will occur in the near future. Advances in the spatial resolution of magnetic resonance imaging (MRI) have allowed us to offer MR enterography in selected patients.

To conclude, CTE is a significant advance in small bowel imaging over SBFT. At our center and many others, CTE has largely replaced SBFT as the first-line small bowel imaging modality in patients with known or suspected CD due to its increased sensitivity in the detection of active small bowel inflammation, ability to detect extraluminal complications, and superior specificity relative to capsule endoscopy.

References

1. Paulsen SR, Huprich JE, Fletcher JG, et al. CT enterography as a diagnostic tool in evaluating small bowel disorders: review of clinical experience with over 700 cases. *Radiographics*. 2006;26(3):641-657.
2. Triester SL, Leighton JA, Leontiadis GI, et al. A meta-analysis of the yield of capsule endoscopy compared to other diagnostic modalities in patients with non-stricturing small bowel Crohn's disease. *Am J Gastroenterol*. 2006;101(5):954-964.
3. Bodily KD, Fletcher JG, Solem CA, et al. Crohn disease: mural attenuation and thickness at contrast-enhanced CT enterography—correlation with endoscopic and histologic findings of inflammation. *Radiology*. 2006;238(2):505-516.
4. Colombel JF, Solem CA, Sandborn WJ, et al. Quantitative measurement and visual assessment of ileal Crohn's disease activity by computed tomography enterography: correlation with endoscopic severity and C reactive protein. *Gut*. 2006;55(11):1561-1567.
5. Solem CA, Loftus EV, Fletcher JG, et al. Small bowel imaging in Crohn's disease: a prospective, blinded, 4-way comparison trial. *Gastrointest Endosc*. 2008;68(2):255-266.
6. Bruining DH, Sidikki H, Fletcher JG, Tremaine WJ, Sandborn WJ, Loftus EV. Prevalence of penetrating disease and extraintestinal manifestations of Crohn's disease detected with CT enterography. *Inflamm Bowel Dis*. 2008;14(12):1701-1706.
7. Higgins PD, Caoili E, Zimmermann M, et al. Computed tomographic enterography adds information to clinical management in small bowel Crohn's disease. *Inflamm Bowel Disease*. 2006;13(3):262-268.
8. Peloquin JM, Pardi DS, Sandborn WJ, et al. Exposure to diagnostic ionizing radiation in a population-based cohort of patients with inflammatory bowel disease (abstract). *Am J Gastroenterol*. 2008;103(8):2015-2022.

24

I Recently Did a Capsule Endoscopy on a Young Patient With Diarrhea. The Colonoscopy, Endoscopy, and Biopsies Were All Normal, but the Capsule Showed Several Erosions Scattered Throughout the Small Bowel. Is This Crohn's Disease?

Jonathan A. Leighton, MD, FACG, AGAF

The diagnosis of small bowel Crohn's disease (CD) can be very challenging because there is no gold standard diagnostic test that automatically makes the diagnosis. One retrospective study followed patients with nonspecific ileal erosions found on ileoscopy during routine colonoscopy for mild alterations in bowel habits.[1] Biopsies showed focal laminal propria edema, mild active inflammation, and crypt disarray. The colon was normal in all patients. The mean length of follow-up was 5.8 years. The study found that 8 patients (29%) developed CD after a mean interval of 3.6 years. In the other 20 patients, the lesions resolved. The conclusion was that most focal ileal erosions in patients with mildly altered bowel habits are idiopathic and clinically insignificant. Presumably, these erosions were caused by some other etiology. The diagnosis of CD can be even more challenging when the inflammation is mild and/or confined only to the small bowel. The diagnosis must be based on a constellation of findings, including the history and physical exam, along with laboratory, radiologic, endoscopic, and pathologic findings (Table 24-1). Chronicity of the inflammation is also important to document before making a definitive diagnosis of CD.

Table 24-1

How Crohn's Disease Is Diagnosed

- Clinical history
- Physical examination
- Laboratory tests
- Endoscopy
- X-ray findings
- Tissue biopsy

Capsule endoscopy (CE) has definitely revolutionized our ability to carefully examine the mucosa of the small bowel. Part of the reason for this is that the vast majority of the small bowel is inaccessible to standard endoscopy. Over the past several years, CE has shown tremendous promise in the evaluation and diagnosis of the small bowel in patients with inflammatory conditions. As a result, it has been studied as an alternative modality for diagnosing small bowel CD. In fact, several prospective studies and a meta-analysis have shown that CE is more sensitive than other endoscopic and radiologic modalities for detecting non-stricturing CD of the small bowel. The capsule endoscope can identify erythema, edema, villous blunting, erosions, ulcerations, and strictures (Figure 24-1). However, while CE is very good at detecting inflammation in the small bowel, including erosions, it is extremely important to remember that this finding is not diagnostic for CD. Furthermore, there is evidence to suggest that up to 13% of normal, asymptomatic individuals can have mucosal breaks and other minor lesions of the small bowel detected by CE.[2]

When one finds erosions in the small bowel, there are definitely other etiologies that must be considered. Other causes include celiac disease, infection, ischemia, radiation injury, and autoimmune diseases, as well as immunodeficiency-related, allergic, and drug-induced etiologies. For example, non-steroidal anti-inflammatory drug (NSAID) enteropathy, also known as diaphragm disease, is common and should be excluded before a diagnosis of occult small bowel CD is considered.[3] While NSAID enteropathy typically presents with circumferential ulcerations and thin ring-like diaphragms, it can also mimic CD (Figure 24-2). Therefore, capsule endoscopic findings of mucosal lesions of the small bowel alone are not sufficient for a diagnosis of CD. It remains unclear as to whether the lesions detected by CE in NSAID enteropathy can be reliably distinguished from those due to CD. When NSAID enteropathy is in the differential diagnosis, the chronicity of the lesions also needs to be established prior to the diagnosis of CD.

Future studies need to determine the specificity of the CE finding of small bowel erosions for CD. A minimum standard terminology system for CE has been compiled, but has not been universally adopted.[4] Recently, a standard terminology system has been developed for CD, along with a capsule-scoring index based on villous edema, ulceration, and/or stenosis.[5] It is critical that such a standardized scoring system be utilized by clinical investigators carrying out CE so that the data from future trials are standardized and comparable. It will also be important to develop a system for classifying the extent and

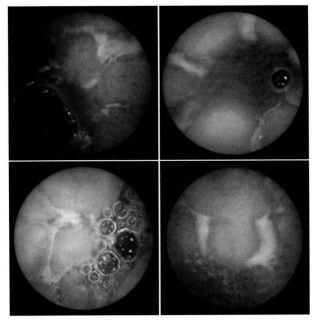

Figure 24-1. Examples of Crohn's disease identified on capsule endoscopy.

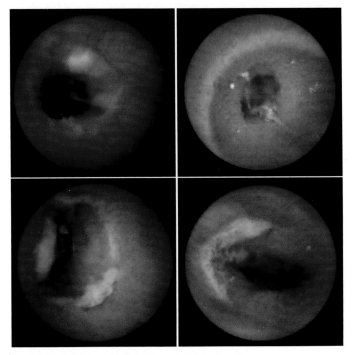

Figure 24-2. Typical findings of NSAID enteropathy.

Table 24-2

Potential Value of a Standardized Scoring System

- Provides an aid to diagnosis and a measure of mucosal damage
- Combined with other clinical parameters, could provide a threshold for differential diagnosis
- Minimizes the subjective nature of assessing disease activity
- Assists in determining appropriate patient management
- Facilitates communication and standardization for assessing disease states
- Helps monitor drug therapy effectiveness

---

severity of inflammatory lesions seen on CE in normal individuals, and to develop criteria for the diagnosis of CD (Table 24-2).

One of the main limitations of CE in the assessment of small bowel CD is the lack of uniform criteria for diagnosing CD, and the inability to allow for tissue acquisition or therapeutic intervention. Efforts to improve biopsy capabilities and remote control capabilities with the capsule are ongoing. It may be possible to develop capsules that will enable physicians to examine the lesion in greater depth, or to take tissue biopsies. However, such capabilities will not be available in the near future. In the meantime, it is important to complement CE with other modalities to establish a diagnosis of CD. Enteroscopy is extremely important. Enteroscopy, such as push enteroscopy or balloon-assisted enteroscopy using the single or double-balloon technique, enables a larger part of the small bowel mucosa to be seen. In addition, enteroscopy allows for the biopsy of lesions. In addition to pathology, laboratory tests including inflammatory markers and serology may also prove beneficial in aiding with the diagnosis. Radiologic tests such as the small bowel follow-through, computed tomography enterography (CTE), and magnetic resonance (MR) enterography can also help in the diagnosis.

In summary, there is no single diagnostic test for small bowel CD. As a result, erosions in the small bowel are not always CD. One needs to consider other potential causes, do appropriate complementary diagnostic tests, and also establish chronicity. Only then can one be more certain of a final diagnosis of CD.

References

1. Goldstein NS. Isolated ileal erosions in patients with mildly altered bowel habits: a follow-up study of 28 patients. *Am J Clin Pathol.* 2006;125(6):838-846.
2. Goldstein JL, Eisen GM, Lewis B, Gralnek IM, Zlotnick S, Fort JG. Video capsule endoscopy to prospectively assess small bowel injury with celecoxib, naproxen plus omeprazole, and placebo. *Clin Gastroenterol Hepatol.* 2005;3(2):133-141.
3. Yousfi MM, De Petris G, Leighton JA, et al. Diaphragm disease after use of nonsteroidal anti-inflammatory agents: first report of diagnosis with capsule endoscopy. *J Clin Gastroenterol.* 2004;38(8):686-691.
4. Korman LY, Delvaux M, Gay G, et al. Capsule endoscopy structured terminology (CEST): proposal of a standardized and structured terminology for reporting capsule endoscopy procedures. *Endoscopy.* 2005;37(10):951-959.
5. Gralnek IM, Defranchis R, Seidman E, Leighton JA, Legnani P, Lewis BS. Development of a capsule endoscopy scoring index for small bowel mucosal inflammatory change. *Aliment Pharmacol Ther.* 2008;27(2):146-154.

HOW DO YOU DIAGNOSE POUCHITIS?

Bo Shen, MD, FACG

DO YOU HAVE TO SCOPE EVERYONE?

Patients with pouchitis typically present with an increased frequency of loose stools, urgency, incontinence, nocturnal seepage, abdominal cramps, and pelvic discomfort. However, these symptoms are not specific for pouchitis. Patients with other inflammatory (eg, Crohn's disease [CD] of the pouch and cuffitis) and functional (eg, irritable pouch syndrome [IPS]) disorders of the pouch can also have similar presentations. In addition, these symptoms can be present in patients with surgical complications such as pouch sinus, pouch leak, and anastomotic stricture. In fact, approximately 50% of the patients with these symptoms indeed have endoscopy-proven pouchitis.

Pouch endoscopy is the most valuable tool for the diagnosis and differential diagnosis of pouchitis. A careful pouch endoscopy with mucosal biopsy could achieve the following goals:

- Assess and grade the severity, distribution, and extent of mucosal inflammation of the pouch

- Detect features suggestive of cuffitis (ie, inflammation of the cuff) or CD (eg, discrete ulcers and inflammation of the afferent limb with or without pouch inlet or distal small bowel strictures)

- Identify anatomic abnormalities related to the surgery, such as anastomotic or pouch inlet strictures, pouch sinus, and fistulae

- Perform surveillance for dysplastic lesions in the cuff or pouch

- Deliver endoscopic therapy, such as polypectomy, balloon stricture dilation with or without intra-lesional injection of long-active corticosteroid, cauterization of bleeding lesions, and removal of pouch bezoars

Ideally, pouch endoscopy with biopsy should be performed in all patients with active symptoms in order to make the correct diagnosis. Previous studies have shown a combined assessment of symptoms, and endoscopic and histologic inflammation is necessary to make an accurate diagnosis.[1] However, under certain circumstances, empiric antibiotic therapy with metronidazole or ciprofloxacin can be initiated without performance of pouch endoscopy. If patients respond to antibiotic therapy, a diagnosis of pouchitis or proximal small bowel bacterial overgrowth can be entertained.

WHO IS AT GREATEST RISK?

Risk factors for the development of pouchitis have been extensively studied. There are some variations in identified risk factors among different studies. Genetic polymorphisms such as those of interleukin-1 (IL-1) receptor antagonist and NOD2/CARD15 may increase the risk for pouchitis. Reported risk factors for pouchitis also include a non-carrier status of tumor-necrosis factor (TNF) allele 2, extensive ulcerative colitis (UC), backwash ileitis, proctocolectomy thrombocytosis, extra-intestinal manifestations (especially primary sclerosing cholangitis [PSC]), the presence of perinuclear anti-neutrophil cytoplasmic antibodies (p-ANCA), being a nonsmoker, and the use of non-steroidal anti-inflammatory drugs (NSAIDs). In addition to p-ANCA, the presence of serologic markers, anti-*Saccharomyces cerevisiae* antibodies (ASCA), a CD-related antigen from *Pseudomonas flourescens* and the outer membrane porin C (OmpC) of *Escherichia coli* in patients with preoperative indeterminate colitis (IC) appears to be associated with persistent inflammation of the pouch after restorative proctocolectomy. Acute and chronic pouchitis may have different risk factors.

WHEN IS IT CROHN'S DISEASE?

CD of the pouch can occur after restorative proctocolectomy with ileal pouch-anal anastomosis (IPAA) intentionally performed in a selected group of patients with Crohn's colitis with no previous small intestinal or perianal disease. CD is also inadvertently found in colectomy specimens of patients with a preoperative diagnosis of UC or IC. De novo CD of the pouch may develop weeks to years after IPAA for UC, and a reassessment of the proctocolectomy specimens may show no evidence of CD. Reported cumulative frequencies of CD of the pouch range from 2.7% to 13%. Clinically, CD of the pouch can be classified into inflammatory, fibrostenotic, or fistulizing phenotypes (Figure 25-1). Clinical presentation of CD of the pouch can overlap with that of pouchitis or other inflammatory and non-inflammatory conditions of the pouch. For example, increased stool frequency, urgency, and abdominal cramps can be presenting symptoms in CD of the pouch, as well as in pouchitis and cuffitis. Symptoms of bloating, nausea, and vomiting can be seen in both fibrostenotic CD of the pouch and anastomotic strictures associated with the pouch surgery. Although there are no specific symptoms or signs of CD of the pouch, fistula drainage, weight loss, anemia, and low-grade fever are more often seen in patients with CD of the pouch.

In a broad sense, disease activity of CD of the pouch may not be limited to the pouch per se. CD in patients with ileal pouches can occur in any part of the gastrointestinal (GI) tract. The diagnosis of CD of the pouch often rests on a combined assessment of symptoms, endoscopy, histology, and radiography. Endoscopic features suggestive of CD of the pouch include the presence of afferent limb ulcers and/or stricture in the setting of ulcerated stricture of the pouch inlet and the presence of ulcers or stricture in other parts of the small bowel in the absence of NSAID use. Morphologic characteristics of ulcers in the pouch were not reliable for the distinction between CD of the pouch and pouchitis. It is important to differentiate NSAID-induced ileitis/pouchitis from CD ileitis and backwash ileitis with diffuse pouchitis. Typically, CD ileitis is characterized by discrete ulcers in the distal neo-terminal ileum (> 10 cm beyond the pouch inlet) and ulcerated stricture at the pouch inlet. In contrast, backwash ileitis with diffuse pouchitis is characterized by

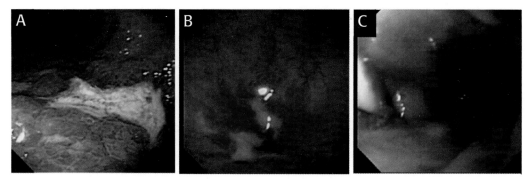

Figure 25-1. Endoscopic view of inflammatory (A), fibrostenotic (B), and fistulizing (C, with seton in place) Crohn's disease of the pouch.

the presence of continuous endoscopic and histologic inflammation from the pouch to the distal neo-terminal ileum (typically within 10 cm of pouch inlet) with widely patent pouch inlet. It is also important to distinguish surgery-associated stricture and fistulizing complications from fibrostenotic or fistulizing CD. However, these distinctions can be difficult to make. In clinical practice, CD of the pouch should be suspected if a patient develops de novo fistula more than 6 to 12 months after ileostomy take-down in the absence of postoperative leak, abscess, and sepsis. Cuffitis refractory to topical therapy with anti-inflammatory agents should raise suspicion for CD-associated cuffitis. Imaging studies such as pelvic magnetic resonance imaging (MRI) or examination under general anesthesia often yield anatomic abnormalities outside of the cuff such as fistulae, leaks, and even abscesses. The presence of histologic evidence of granulomas or pyloric gland metaplasia would also suggest a diagnosis of CD.[2]

WHEN IS IT POSTSURGICAL COMPLICATIONS?

Restorative proctocolectomy with IPAA is a technically demanding complex procedure. Short- and long-term surgical complications are common. These complications include anastomotic leaks (at the pouch-anal anastomosis, the tip of the "J", and the body of the pouch along the staple line), pelvic sepsis (one of the most common causes for pouch failure), abscess, pouch sinus, pouch fistula, strictures (at anastomosis or pouch outlet stricture, mid-pouch, pouch inlet, or afferent limb stricture), afferent and efferent limb syndrome (partial obstruction of afferent or efferent limbs), infertility, male and female sexual dysfunction, portal vein thrombi, pouch herniation or intussusception, pouch prolapse (mucosal versus full-thickness prolapse), twisted pouch or volvulus, dysfunctional megapouch, trapped ovary syndrome, and pouch bleeding.

It is particularly important to distinguish surgery-related strictures and fistulae from ones related to CD. CD-related strictures or fistulae are often associated with other inflammatory features of the afferent limb or pouch. In addition, timing and locations of the fistulae are the key. For example, the occurrence of a fistula without initial anastomotic leak, particularly when it develops more than 6 to 12 months after ileostomy take-down, can be a harbinger for CD. Fistula below the anastomosis level can result from CD or cryptoglandar sepsis. The latter occurs in patients with underlying UC with late spontaneous development of a fistula, which sometimes is difficult to distinguish from CD. However, recurrent, multiple, complex, or anovaginal features of fistulae would suggest a diagnosis of CD, especially if other perianal lesions exist.

Pouch-vaginal fistula (PVF) is a unique and yet common condition with ileal pouches, and it is one of the most common causes for pouch failure. PVF can develop early (< 6 months after IPAA) or late (> 12 months after IPAA). PVF can present at, below, or above the anastomosis, and it presents as a simple or complex fistulae with multiple fistulous tracts. A diagnosis of CD should be suspected in patients with PVF if they have: 1) a pre-operative diagnosis of CD, IC, or IC favoring CD; 2) the presence of a fistula 6 to 12 months after IPAA in the absence of pelvic abscess or pelvic sepsis, although there is no consensus in the literature regarding the cut-off time of occurrence of a PVF for the diagnosis of CD; 3) the presence of a complex PVF; 4) the presence of a PVF outside of the pouch-anal anas-tomosis; or 5) concurrent ulcerated lesions in the small bowel or afferent limb.

WHAT IS AN "IRRITABLE" POUCH?

IPS is a functional disorder in patients with ileal pouches. It is considered as a unique form of irritable bowel syndrome (IBS). The etiology and pathophysiology are not clear. It may be attributed to psychosocial factors, visceral hypersensitivity, and enterochromaf-fin cell hyperplasia of the pouch mucosa. Clinical presentations of pouchitis, cuffitis, and IPS often overlap. Common symptoms include increased stool frequency and decreased stool consistency, urgency, and abdominal pain. Some of the patients may respond to oral antibiotic therapy, suggesting that proximal small bowel bacterial overgrowth may contribute to patients' symptoms. Currently, IPS is a diagnosis of exclusion based on the presence of symptoms of increased frequency of bowel movements with a change in stool consistency, abdominal pain, and perianal or pelvic discomfort in the absence of endo-scopic and histologic inflammation. It is important to exclude celiac disease, and lactose or fructose intolerance.

References

1. Shen B, Fazio VW, Remzi FH, et al. Comprehensive evaluation of inflammatory and non-inflammatory sequelae of ileal pouch-anal anastomosis. *Am J Gastroenterol.* 2005;100(1):93-101.
2. Shen B, Remzi FH, Lavery IC, Lashner BA, Fazio VW. A proposed classification of ileal pouch disorders and associated complications after restorative proctocolectomy for ulcerative colitis. *Clin Gastroenterol Hepatol.* 2008;6(2):145-148.

HOW DO YOU TREAT POUCHITIS?

Kim L. Isaacs, MD, PhD, AGAF

Total abdominal colectomy with ileal-pouch anal anastomosis (IPAA) has become the main surgical alternative for medically refractory ulcerative colitis (UC), UC with dysplasia, and familial adenomatous polyposis (FAP) over the past 2 decades. It is estimated that up to 60% of patients who undergo this procedure for UC will experience at least one episode of pouchitis (Figure 26-1).[1] Patients with FAP rarely undergo this complication of IPAA. Patients typically present with an increased stool frequency, pelvic discomfort, urgency, and, occasionally, stool leakage and rectal bleeding. Although the etiology of pouchitis is unknown, most studies suggest that there is an abnormal immune response to the pouch microflora, which leads to both acute and chronic inflammation. Approaches to the treatment of pouchitis have involved the manipulation of both the pouch microflora and the mucosal immune system.

In a patient presenting with symptoms of pouchitis, the first thing that should be done is to confirm the diagnosis with an endoscopic exam of the ileal pouch.[2] Motility disturbances of the pouch (irritable pouch syndrome [IPS]) and inflammation of the cuff (cuffitis) can mimic symptoms of pouchitis, but require different therapies (Table 26-1). In addition, it is not uncommon for patients, initially felt to have UC prior to colectomy, to develop inflammatory changes above the pouch more consistent with Crohn's disease (CD). The approach to therapy in this population is to use treatment regimens directed at the CD and not the pouchitis. The second issue to explore is the use of non-steroidal anti-inflammatory drugs (NSAIDs). NSAID use can present a picture in the ileal pouch suggestive of pouchitis. This entity responds to discontinuing NSAIDs.[3]

Once pouchitis is established, the next step is to define the process as acute pouchitis, acute recurrent pouchitis, or chronic pouchitis. If this is the first bout of pouchitis, this distinction may not be possible, but will evolve over time.

In a patient presenting with a first episode of acute pouchitis, antibiotics are the mainstay of therapy, although optimal treatment regimens remain to be defined. My practice is to start with a metronidazole 500 mg bid (twice a day) and, if not tolerated, then switch to a ciprofloxacin 500 mg bid. Small, controlled clinical trials have been performed demonstrating the benefit of short-term treatment with metronidazole and ciprofloxacin, with some suggestion that ciprofloxacin had fewer side effects.[4] Metronidazole therapy has also been compared in a controlled fashion to budesonide enemas with similar efficacy

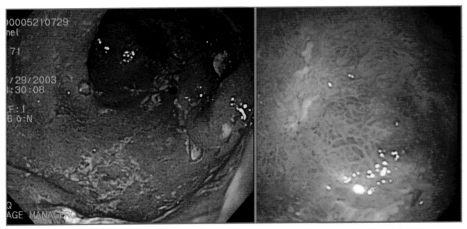

Figure 26-1. Pouchitis, endoscopically, is characterized by granularity, friability, and ulceration of the ileal pouch.

Table 26-1

Differential Diagnosis of Pouchitis

- Idiopathic pouchitis
- Crohn's disease
- Irritable pouch syndrome
- Cytomegalovirus infection
- *Clostridia difficile* infection
- Cuffitis
- Anastomotic stricture
- NSAID effect
- Ischemia
- Pelvic floor dyssynergia
- Anal sphincter dysfunction

---

reported. Uncontrolled studies have reported beneficial responses in patients with pouchitis to erythromycin, tetracycline, rifaximin, and amoxicillin/clavulanate.[1] Patients who cannot tolerate the systemic side effects of metronidazole at a dose of 750 to 1500 mg/day may tolerate a low dose of metronidazole at 70 to 300 mg/day given topically bid into the pouch in the form of a formulated suppository or a vaginal gel. With the first bout of pouchitis, or in patients with recurrent acute pouchitis that is infrequent, I typically treat for 14 days. The length of treatment varies in the reported controlled and uncontrolled trials from as few as 7 days up to 30 days. Rifaximin and other non-absorbable antibiotics have a theoretic advance of little or no systemic absorption leading to systemic side effects. Although large scale, rigorous, controlled trials have not been performed with rifaximin, I will use this as an alternative to metronidazole and ciprofloxacin in patients who are poorly tolerant of these drugs. The doses that have been used in clinical trials and open label studies range from 400 mg tid (three times a day) to 1 gram bid.

Chronic pouchitis is much more of a management problem in many patients. In patients who respond readily to a course of antibiotics but develop recurrent symptoms off of the antibiotics, the common practice is to treat chronically with the antibiotic that induced a resolution of the symptoms. Some patients are able to maintain remission on lower doses of antibiotics than on that needed to induce remission. Metronidazole is associated with more short-term and long-term side effects than is ciprofloxacin, limiting its use chronically. Short-term side effects include nausea, vomiting, abdominal pain, metallic taste in the mouth, headache, and rash. Peripheral neuropathy can occur with long-term use and may be irreversible. The most common antibiotic regimens used for chronic pouchitis are ciprofloxacin 250 to 500 mg/day and metronidazole 500 mg/day. Patients on maintenance antibiotics who lose response may respond to rotating antibiotics in 1 to 3 week intervals (eg, 3 weeks of metronidazole, followed by 3 weeks of ciprofloxacin, and then 3 weeks of rifaximin.) Short-term combination antibiotics such as ciprofloxacin/metronidazole or ciprofloxacin/rifaximin may also re-induce remission in patients who lose response to a single antibiotic.

With concerns about the chronic use of systemically absorbed antibiotics in patients with chronic pouchitis, alternative approaches to management should be considered. Non-absorbable antibiotics such as rifaximin may play a role, but they have only been studied adequately in a controlled fashion as combination therapy with ciprofloxacin in patients with chronic refractory pouchitis. Probiotics have received much attention as a means of altering the pouch flora and maintaining remission in chronic pouchitis. Oral probiotics containing strains of lactobacilli, bifidobacteria, and streptococcus (VSL#3; Sigma-Tau Pharmaceuticals, Inc., Gaithersburg, MD) have the most trial data to support their use.[5,6] Open label clinical experience is encouraging. Patients are first treated with an antibiotic course to induce remission, and then the probiotic combination is added and administered chronically after the antibiotic course is completed. I will try this approach in patients with chronic pouchitis who are willing to take a daily probiotic supplement. My practice is to give 1 packet of VSL#3 tid, or a twice-daily dosing of an alternative probiotic that contains multiple strains of probiotic organisms.

If antibiotics or antibiotic/probiotic combinations are not successful in managing pouchitis symptoms, the diagnosis should again be questioned. In patients who clearly have continued active pouchitis, budesonide may play a role in treating active inflammation. Two mg budesonide enemas have demonstrated efficacy in clinical trials, but are not readily available in the United States. An alternative is to start 9 mg/day of oral budesonide and taper down to the lowest dose possible to manage symptoms. These patients will require attention to bone health with calcium and vitamin D supplementation, as well as with monitoring bone density. Topical therapy with mesalamine has not been found to be routinely effective in the treatment of acute or chronic pouchitis.

In patients who continue to have refractory pouchitis, there are anecdotal reports of the efficacy of immunomodulators such as 6-mercaptopurine (6-MP)/azathioprine and infliximab.[2] These agents have not been subject to randomized controlled trials. However, since the alternative of removing the pouch and creating an end ileostomy is not acceptable to many patients, I have used these agents with some success. The dosing is the same as what would be used to treat CD—1 to 1.5 mg/kg of 6-MP, 2 to 2.5 mg/kg of azathioprine, and 5 mg/kg of infliximab per 2 months.

Overall, pouchitis is a common and often frustrating disease entity to treat. Accurate diagnosis and initial treatment with antibiotics should be undertaken. For patients with chronic pouchitis, long-term low-dose antibiotics or antibiotics followed by probiotics should be considered. In patients who continue to have problems, oral budesonide may control symptoms. In patients who continue to have refractory disease, immunosuppression or immunomodulation with 6-MP, azathioprine, or infliximab can be considered. Rarely, the patient may require resection of the ileal pouch with the creation of an end-ileostomy.

References

1. Pardi DS, Sandborn WJ. Systematic review: the management of pouchitis. *Aliment Pharmacol Ther.* 2006;23(8):1087-1096.
2. Pardi DS, Shen B. Endoscopy in the management of patients after ileal pouch surgery for ulcerative colitis. *Endoscopy.* 2008;40(6):529-533.
3. Shen B, Fazio VW, Remzi FH. Effect of withdrawal of nonsteroidal anti-inflammatory drug use on ileal pouch disorders. *Digestive Diseases and Sciences.* 2007;52(12):3321-3328.
4. Shen B, Achkar JP, Lashner BA, et al. A randomized clinical trial of ciprofloxacin and metronidazole to treat acute pouchitis. *Inflamm Bowel Dis.* 2001;7(4):301-305.
5. Gionchetti PP. Oral bacteriotherapy as maintenance treatment in patients with chronic pouchitis: a double-blind, placebo-controlled trial. *Gastroenterology.* 2000;119(2):594-587.
6. Gionchetti PP, Rizzello F, Morselli C, et al. High-dose probiotics for the treatment of active pouchitis diseases of the colon and rectum. 2007;50(12):2075-2084.

MY PARTNER TELLS ME THAT "SEROLOGY 7" PROFILES CAN PREDICT WHICH CROHN'S DISEASE PATIENTS WILL PROGRESS RAPIDLY. SHOULD I ORDER THIS FOR ALL OF MY NEWLY DIAGNOSED CROHN'S DISEASE PATIENTS? ARE THERE ADDITIONAL CLINICAL OR GENETIC FACTORS THAT IDENTIFY A HIGH-RISK GROUP?

Marla C. Dubinsky, MD

Individuals with Crohn's disease (CD) show a wide variation in the way they present and progress over time. Some patients present with mild disease activity and do well with generally safe and mild medications. Many, however, exhibit more severe disease with an impaired quality of life, continued active gastrointestinal (GI) symptoms, and the eventual development of disease complications requiring surgery. Current and emerging potent therapies that target the immune system have helped decrease symptoms and appear to decrease the need for surgery. However, these therapies have increased the potential risk for serious side effects such as infection and malignancy. Being able to define at the time of diagnosis those individuals most likely to require aggressive medical therapy will provide the doctor and patient information to better decide which therapy is best.

Subsets of patients with differing immune responses to microbial antigens have been described: antibodies to the *Escherichia coli* (*E. coli*) outer-membrane porin C (OmpC), as well as anti-*Saccharomyces cerevisiae* (ASCA) and autoantigens (ie, perinuclear anti-neutrophil antibody [pANCA]). A novel immune response, anti-flagellin (anti-CBir1), has been identified in approximately 50% of CD patients and has been suggested to represent a unique subgroup of CD patients.

Both genetic and immune markers have been examined as possible predictors of a more aggressive disease course. The original NOD2 studies found an association between NOD2 and small bowel fibrostenosing disease.[1] Subsequent studies, however, have suggested that serological immune markers (antibodies driven by specific microbial antigens), not NOD2, may be more important predictors of disease complications. It appears that NOD2 is associated with small bowel disease location only. On the other hand, the immune responses (ASCA in particular) have been shown to be associated with fibrostenosing, internal penetrating small bowel disease, and small bowel surgery. The research suggests that the presence (number of markers) and magnitude (antibody level) of immune responses to microbial antigens is significantly associated with more aggressive disease phenotypes.[2] This concept was adopted and applied to a large CD cohort investigating a novel panel of anti-glycan antibodies, and similar associations were found with disease behavior. In theory, higher levels of immune responses may reflect the degree of genetically predisposed mucosal dysregulation characteristic of CD leading to a loss of ability to tolerate specific bacteria. Moreover, data now exist that links seroreactivity to microbial antigens to underlying genetically determined innate immune defects (NOD2).[3]

A recent prospective study conducted in a large pediatric cohort demonstrated that the time to develop a disease complication in children is significantly faster in the presence of immune responses, thereby predicting disease progression to more aggressive disease phenotypes among pediatric CD patients. Those patients positive for at least 2 immune responses (ASCA, anti-OmpC, or anti-CBir1) progressed to internal penetrating and/or fibrostenosing disease faster than those negative for all or positive for only 1 antibody.[4] The group positive for all 3 antibodies demonstrated the most rapid disease progression. These preliminary findings suggest that immune markers may indeed be predictive of a more aggressive disease course. However, larger prospective studies in both children and adults need to be conducted to make a more definitive conclusion about the ability of genetics or serum biomarkers to predict natural history.

Clinical factors at diagnosis have also been described in association with disabling or complicated CD.[5] When it comes to clinical factors, the initial requirement for steroid use, an age at diagnosis below 40 years, and the presence of perianal disease at diagnosis have been shown to be independently associated with subsequent 5-year disabling CD. Longitudinal studies are currently underway to evaluate which factors (clinical, genetic, and immune) or a combination thereof will predict the natural history of the disease to help stratify patients at diagnosis. Thus, choosing patients whose risk of rapid disease progression to disease complications outweighs the risk of the individual therapies is critical in moving forward in developing the most appropriate therapeutic paradigms.

Immune marker testing, as offered by the current inflammatory bowel disease (IBD) Serology 7, may serve as an additional tool to help communicate with patients the risk of disease progression. When clinical symptoms and the use of steroids drive the decision to start immunomodulation like 6-mercaptopurine (6-MP) or azathioprine, then immune response testing may not add anything to the therapeutic strategy. However, when the decision is difficult for patients and physicians, the results of the immune markers testing may help drive the decision in one direction or another. The real question will be when deciding on whom to use a biologic therapy at the time of presentation, and I do not think that the current data is convincing enough to drive that level of decision making. The longitudinal studies will certainly help answer that question. I think knowledge of the immune profiles for patients is helpful and can be another piece of the puzzle when managing both the short- and long-term course of patients with CD. Since the uncertain nature of the disease is a major concern to our patients, the ability to communicate risk and predict potential outcomes is something that is viewed as helpful to our patients. The science is progressing rapidly in this field, and clinicians now have the opportunity to begin to integrate our understanding of the immune and genetic differences of our patients into treatment decision making.

References

1. Abreu MT, Taylor KD, Lin YC, et al. Mutations in NOD2 are associated with fibrostenosing disease in patients with Crohn's disease. *Gastroenterology*. 2002;123(3):679-688.
2. Mow WS, Vasiliauskas EA, Lin YC, et al. Association of antibody responses to microbial antigens and complications of small bowel Crohn's disease. *Gastroenterology*. 2004;126(2):414-424.
3. Devlin SM, Yang H, Ippoliti A, et al. NOD2 Variants and antibody response to microbial antigens in Crohn's disease patients and their unaffected relatives. *Gastroenterology*. 2007;132(2):576-586.
4. Dubinsky MC, Lin YC, Dutridge D, et al. Serum immune responses predict rapid disease progression among children with Crohn's disease: immune responses predict disease progression. *Am J Gastroenterol*. 2006;101(2):360-367.
5. Beaugerie L, Seksik P, Nion-Larmurier I, Gendre JP, Cosnes J. Predictors of Crohn's disease. *Gastroenterology*. 2006;130(3):650-656.

DO ANY MEDICATIONS SLOW THE PROGRESSION OF PRIMARY SCLEROSING CHOLANGITIS?

Marshall M. Kaplan, MD, MACP

Currently, there is no effective treatment for primary sclerosing cholangitis (PSC). Although ursodiol (ursodeoxycholic acid, UDCA) decreases serum levels of alkaline phosphatase, alanine aminotransferase (ALT), and aspartate aminotransferase (AST), it does not slow the progression of PSC. UDCA does not prolong survival or prevent the development of cirrhosis or other complications of PSC in the dose that is effective in the treatment of primary biliary cirrhosis (13 to 15 mg/kg body weight per day).[1] The only study that was of adequate duration to assess survival and included enough patients clearly showed that UDCA had no beneficial effect on survival, symptoms, serum bilirubin levels, liver histology, or the development of cirrhosis and portal hypertension (Figure 28-1).[1] It is possible that a higher dose of UDCA may be effective, but there is no proof of this. Several studies have used higher doses (20 mg/kg and 25 to 30 mg/kg body weight per day, respectively) and reported greater improvement in liver enzyme tests.[2] However, these studies included few patients and were of too short duration to assess survival. The latter study also reported an improvement in the Mayo risk score, a mathematical model that is used to predict survival in PSC.[2] It led to a National Institute of Health (NIH)-funded placebo-controlled multicenter study of a higher UDCA dose (28 to 30 mg/kg body weight per day). Unfortunately, this placebo-controlled trial involving 150 patients had to be stopped early.[3] Patients randomized to UDCA did worse than those on placebo. Patients on UDCA were significantly more likely to reach the primary endpoints selected at the start of the study (namely death, referral for liver transplantation, and the development of esophageal varices).[3] The reasons for this unexpected outcome were unclear. The investigators suggested that high-dose UDCA be restricted to patients in clinical trials.

One problem in finding effective treatment for PSC is that it may be a group of diseases rather than one disease, similar to chronic hepatitis and colitis. For example, there appears to be an autoimmune variant of sclerosing cholangitis whose etiology and treatment is

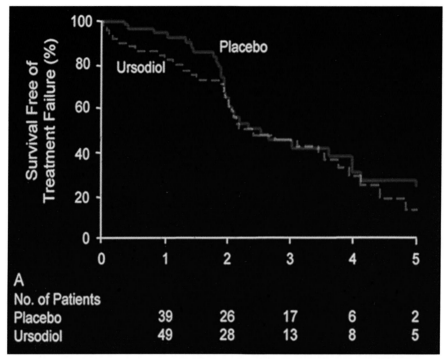

Figure 28-1. Survival free of treatment failure in PSC patients on ursodiol or placebo. Copyright © 1997 Massachusettes Medical Society. All rights reserved.

different from that of typical PSC.[4,5] Although elevated immunoglobulin G4 (IgG4) levels are found in some of these patients, I have not found elevated IgG4 levels in the majority of patients with autoimmune cholangitis whom I have seen. I believe that the response to treatment with immunosuppressive drugs such as prednisone and methotrexate (MTX) is a better way to identify them, particularly since prednisone and/or MTX may be effective treatment for these patients.[4,5]

There is one additional factor that must be considered before UDCA and immunosuppressive drugs are discarded as effective treatment for PSC—the difficulty in designing and performing treatment trials in PSC. The etiology of PSC is unknown. Therefore, the use of any drug is an educated guess. In addition, PSC appears to be more complicated than other liver diseases. PSC may be caused by multiple interacting pathogenetic factors such as impaired host defenses and chronic infection. There are multiple bile duct strictures in PSC that obstruct bile flow. These may cause chronic infections that are difficult to treat. Last and perhaps most important, PSC is usually diagnosed late in its course. The diagnosis of PSC is based on unequivocal cholangiographic abnormalities, typically multiple bile duct strictures and dilatations. These changes are most often caused by scarred bile ducts. Scarring is a late manifestation in inflammatory diseases and may define a population that has irreversible damage and is already untreatable. The ability to diagnose PSC before bile duct scarring occurs would greatly advance our ability to find effective treatment.

References

1. Lindor KD, Mayo Primary Sclerosing Cholangitis-Ursodeoxycholic Acid Study Group. Ursodeoxycholic acid for primary sclerosing cholangitis. *N Engl J Med.* 1997;336(10):691-695.
2. Harnois DM, Angulo P, Jorgensen RA, LaRusso NF, Lindor KD. High-dose ursodeoxycholic acid as a therapy for patients with primary sclerosing cholangitis. *Am J Gastroenterology.* 2001;96(1):1558-1562.
3. Lindor KD, Enders FB, Schmoll JA, et al. Randomized, double-blind controlled trial of high-dose ursodeoxycholic acid (UDCA) for primary sclerosing cholangitis. *Hepatology.* 2008;48(suppl):LB2.
4. Bjornnson E, Chari ST, Smyrk TC, Lindor KD. Immunoglobulin G4 associated cholangitis; description of an emerging clinical entity based on review of the literature. *Hepatology.* 2007;45(6):1547-1554.
5. Sekhon JS, Chung RT, Epstein M, Kaplan MM. Steroid-responsive (autoimmune) sclerosing cholangitis. *Dig Dis Sci.* 2005;50(10):1839-1843.

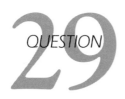

WHAT IS THE BEST APPROACH TO DOSING CYCLOSPORINE FOR SEVERE ULCERATIVE COLITIS? CAN INFLIXIMAB BE USED BEFORE CYCLOSPORINE DOSING? CAN CYCLOSPORINE BE USED BEFORE INFLIXIMAB?

Seamus J. Murphy, PhD, MRCP and Asher Kornbluth, MD

Patients with persistent severe colitis after 7 to 10 days of high-dose intravenous (IV) steroids are unlikely to respond to continued steroid therapy and should be offered IV cyclosporine, infliximab, or surgery.[1,2] Quality of life following cyclosporine use may be better than following colectomy,[3] but there are 2 important preconditions for cyclosporine use: it should only be used in those centers where cyclosporine drug levels can be determined readily, and where gastroenterologists and surgeons experienced with its use are available to monitor patients. Patients are informed of the risks and benefits of colectomy by our surgical colleagues, and cyclosporine is offered as an alternative to infliximab or surgery. Data comparing cyclosporine to infliximab in this situation are not available. We tend to use cyclosporine since 80% of patients will respond to this treatment, will usually do so within 3 to 7 days, and failure to do so indicates the need for surgery. The time required for infliximab to demonstrate effectiveness in this situation is unknown. Furthermore, we have had extensive experience with the use of cyclosporine for this indication for over 20 years, and we have an "exit strategy," whereby patients are either in remission after a 6-month course of oral cyclosporine in conjunction with 6-mercaptopurine (6-MP) or azathioprine, or they undergo colectomy.

Contraindications to cyclosporine use include active infection, uncontrolled hypertension, renal insufficiency, and unreliable patients (frequent physician visits are required following discharge from hospital). Persistent fevers, even if low grade, should prompt a computed tomography (CT) scan of the abdomen and pelvis to exclude the possibility of a sealed or free perforation. Renal function must be monitored closely and may be calculated using the Modification of Diet in Renal Disease (MDRD) equation, which is based on serum creatinine, age, and gender, and provides an estimate of glomerular filtration rate (eGFR). In addition to assessing baseline renal function, serum cholesterol and magnesium should be checked. Low levels of either increase the risk of neurotoxicity, including seizures. Patients with low levels of cholesterol (cholesterol < 120 mg/dL or 3 mmol/L) should be started on lower doses of cyclosporine, and cholesterol and cyclosporine levels should be monitored on a daily basis.

In our experience, patients are started on 4 mg/kg/day of cyclosporine as a continuous infusion. However, other groups have advocated lower doses. Van Assche conducted a randomized controlled trial to study the efficacy of cyclosporine 2 mg/kg versus 4 mg/kg, and found no differences in efficacy.[4] However, the serum cyclosporine levels in the 4 mg/kg group were lower than in our experience with 4 mg/kg, so we have continued to prescribe this dose during the IV phase. We generally aim for levels of cyclosporine of 200 to 400 mg/dL, as measured by the monoclonal assay, during the IV phase. For transitioning to oral cyclosporine upon hospital discharge, we double the dose of the IV (ie, approximately 8 mg/kg orally in 2 divided doses), and generally aim for outpatient levels of 100 to 250 mg/dL. In addition, we initiate treatment with 6-MP and begin a weekly steroid taper. Failure to taper the prednisone and cyclosporine by 3 to 6 months is considered a failure. In terms of serious adverse events, our observation has been that these are related to the concomitant use of high-dose steroids (during the initial cyclosporine phase) rather than the serum level of cyclosporine. Nevertheless, the 2 mg/kg dose may be similarly effective, and it may be a safer alternative.

Infliximab has recently emerged as a potential third alternative for steroid refractory patients with UC. This is based on a randomized, double-blind, placebo-controlled study by Jarnerot et al, which demonstrated that a single infliximab infusion reduced the rate of colectomy at 90 days.[5] Long-term outcomes were not reported, and a strategy for long-term management is not known. Nevertheless, we feel that infliximab is a useful option, but we tend to use that in moderate to severe patients, and cyclosporine in severely ill patients. A randomized, controlled trial comparing infliximab with cyclosporine in severe UC is ongoing in Europe.[6]

With both cyclosporine and infliximab available as options in moderate to severe UC, a question to address is whether the sequential use of these agents in the event of the failure of the first agent should be attempted. A second question to address is whether the sequence of their use influences outcome. We believe that the sequential use of these two drugs in either order is not advisable for the following reasons:

- Serum levels of infliximab typically remain elevated for 8 weeks after infusion, so if cyclosporine is given within this period, there is the potential for potent "double" immunosuppression and increased toxicity.
- The half-life of IV cyclosporine is approximately 6 hours, with an elimination time between 10 and 27 hours.

- While cyclosporine may be absent from serum in patients who receive infliximab, the immunosuppressive effects of 2 agents used sequentially in this way remain unknown.

- We recently reviewed our experience with patients with severe colitis who were treated with cyclosporine followed by infliximab (10 patients) or infliximab followed by cyclosporine (9 patients), with either agent being used within 30 days of the other.[7] The remission rates at 1 year, defined as clinical remission and complete taper off corticosteroids, were low in both groups at 40% and 33%, respectively. Durations of remission were 10.4 months and 28.5 months, respectively. Serious adverse events occurred in 3 patients (16%), including one death in this group of 19 patients.

Therefore, our recommendation is that either cyclosporine or infliximab, but not both, should be considered for the patient with severe colitis as an alternative to colectomy.

References

1. Lichtiger S, Present DH, Kornbluth A, et al. Cyclosporine in severe ulcerative colitis refractory to steroid therapy. *N Engl J Med.* 1994;330(26):1841-1845.
2. Kornbluth A, Present DH, Lichtiger S, Hanauer S. Cyclosporin for severe ulcerative colitis: a user's guide. *Am J Gastroenterol.* 1997;92(9):1424-1428.
3. Cohen RD, Brodsky AL, Hanauer SB. A comparison of the quality of life in patients with severe ulcerative colitis after total colectomy versus medical treatment with intravenous cyclosporin. *Inflamm Bowel Dis.* 1999;5(1):1-10.
4. Van Assche G, D'Haens G, Noman M, et al. Randomized, double-blind comparison of 4 mg/kg versus 2 mg/kg intravenous cyclosporine in severe ulcerative colitis. *Gastroenterology.* 2003;125(4):1025-1031.
5. Jarnerot G, Hertervig E, Friis-Liby I, et al. Infliximab as rescue therapy in severe to moderately severe ulcerative colitis: a randomized, placebo-controlled study. *Gastroenterology.* 2005;128(7):1805-1811.
6. GETAID. CYSIF study. Available at: http:www.getaid.org. Accessed January 15, 2009.
7. Maser EA, Deconda D, Lichtiger S, Ullman T, Present DH, Kornbluth A. Cyclosporine and infliximab as rescue therapy for each other in patients with steroid refractory ulcerative colitis. *Clin Gastroenterol Hepatol.* 2008;6(10):1112-1116.

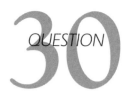

QUESTION

WHEN SHOULD BOWEL REST OR ELEMENTAL FEEDING BE USED IN THE MANAGEMENT OF CROHN'S DISEASE?

Douglas L. Seidner, MD, FACG and Rene Rivera, MD

We commonly use the phrase "if the gut works, use it" when assessing patients that we are asked to see for nutrition support. But the use of this phrase is a topic of debate when referring to adult patients with Crohn's disease (CD), especially during an acute exacerbation. CD has a wide spectrum of severity. While some patients exhibit mildly active disease or disease that is localized to a short segment of bowel and is responsive to medical therapy, others experience frequent moderate to severe exacerbations of their disease that may require multiple hospital admissions and surgical intervention for bowel resection. It is this latter group of patients that are often malnourished and who may benefit from nutrition support. Therefore, the answer to this question depends on several factors, including the extent and activity of disease, whether disease activity is responding to conventional medical therapy, and whether malnutrition is present and, if so, how severe it is. Nutrition can serve as a supportive therapy in patients being managed with medical or surgical treatments, or it can serve as primary therapy in certain clinical situations.[1] We will briefly review the rationale and evidence to help provide guidance in the appropriate use of bowel rest and enteral feeding in the treatment of patients with CD.

CROHN'S DISEASE AND MALNUTRITION

Nutrition should play an integral part in the management of patients with CD due to the high prevalence of protein-calorie malnutrition that is observed in this patient population. It is estimated that 65% to 75% of patients with CD experience malnutrition at some point in their illness.[2] The cause of malnutrition can include the following reasons:
- Reduced oral intake due to abdominal pain, nausea, and diarrhea
- Malabsorption associated with inflamed mucosa or intestinal resection
- Nutrient losses from intestinal inflammation

- Altered metabolism associated with both acute and chronic inflammation
- Drug-nutrient interactions

Therefore, it is important for clinicians to have a high index of suspicion for the presence of malnutrition and to look for signs and symptoms of malnutrition in all patients with CD.

A simple question that we commonly ask is "Have you experienced any unintentional weight loss?" Weight loss and the rate of weight loss have been shown to correlate with morbidity and mortality in hospitalized patients. It is also important to consider specific micronutrient deficiencies that commonly occur in patients with CD as they can result in a decrease in quality of life. These nutrients include calcium, iron, folate, and vitamins D and B12. If there is any evidence of malnutrition, or if its presence is strongly suspected, a thorough nutritional assessment should be performed to accurately diagnose the types and severity of nutrient deficits so that appropriate therapy can be provided.

SELECTING THE ROUTE FOR NUTRITION SUPPORT

The main objective of nutrition intervention is to correct any underlying malnutrition, and then maintain normal levels of both macro- and micro-nutrients. Since CD directly affects the gastrointestinal (GI) tract, the extent and severity of disease activity needs to be considered when selecting the route of nutritional therapy to administer. Having said this, enteral nutrition is always the preferred route to provide nutrients to patients with inflammatory bowel disease (IBD). Circumstances that will prevent or interfere with efforts to use the gut include intractable nausea and vomiting, severe diarrhea or malabsorption, high output enterocutaneous fistula (ECF), and bowel obstruction. Bowel rest is generally not necessary to treat patients with active disease.

One should also be mindful of coexisting digestive disorders that may contribute to the patient's symptoms, and whether enteral feeding will be successful. Lactose intolerance, irritable bowel syndrome (IBS), and bacterial overgrowth in patients with partial bowel obstruction or previous surgery can interfere with food intake if they are not identified and treated.

ENTERAL NUTRITION AS SUPPORTIVE THERAPY

The enteral route is always the preferred method to give nutrition therapy to patients with CD. A healthy, well-balanced diet with no restrictions is encouraged for all patients who can eat food. There should be no difference in the provision of calories from protein, carbohydrates, and fat in patients with CD compared to healthy subjects. However, in patients demonstrating moderate to severe malnutrition, oral intake should be enhanced using nutritional supplements that are high in protein and energy. One should be careful in patients with severe malnutrition since they may be at risk for developing re-feeding syndrome. These patients may need to be hospitalized to allow for the correction of any electrolyte abnormalities prior and during the initiation of nutrition support. If the patient has a limited oral intake due to the fear of eating, anorexia, or nausea, then naso-gastric or naso-jejunal feeding can be considered to help deliver adequate nutrition. In patients with CD strictures, a diet with low-residue is recommended to decrease the incidence of small bowel obstruction.

ENTERAL NUTRITION AS PRIMARY THERAPY

The use of enteral nutrition as a primary modality to treat acute exacerbations of CD stems from the observation that disease activity diminished with bowel rest and malnutrition was commonly associated with this disease. Uncontrolled trials using elemental formulas, which were composed of free amino acids, glucose oligomeres, and low concentrations of fat, resulted in high rates of remission in patients with CD that was refractory to or dependent on corticosteroids.[1] Many of these patients experienced an improvement in nutritional status and were able to decrease or eliminate their dose of corticosteroids. Subsequent randomized trials comparing medical to nutritional therapy found rates of remission at 80% for corticosteroids and 60% for enteral nutrition. While the response rate was not as good as the preliminary uncontrolled trials, the patients who received enteral nutrition still had a better response rate than that seen in the placebo arm of other controlled trials. In addition, the response time for corticosteroids is typically 2 to 3 weeks, while improvement with enteral nutrition can take as long as 4 to 6 weeks. Because of these limitations, we reserve the use of enteral nutrition to adult patients with malnutrition who are responding poorly or develop significant side effects to immunomodulatory therapy. Patients need to be highly motivated as formulas are not as palatable as regular food. They should also be made aware of the slow response rate to this form of medical treatment. Placement of an enteral feeding tube may improve compliance and response rates to this therapy. Finally, even if enteral nutrition leads to disease remission, it does not guarantee maintenance of remission. The relapse rate at 1 year can reach 65% to 100%. However, this is similar to what is seen when other therapies are stopped after treating an acute exacerbation. Patients should be made aware of this, and that pharmacotherapy may be required.

Several hypotheses have been proposed to explain the remission observed with this therapy. These include reductions in antigenic load, alterations in the gut flora, modulation of the intestinal immunophenotype, and improved nutritional status. To date, the exact mechanisms have not been elucidated.

Although an elemental formula was thought to be important in inducing remission in CD, it is now known that there is no difference between this formula, a semi-elemental formula, or a polymeric formula. Low-fat formulas may be potential factors leading to improved efficacy. Therefore, formulas with low fat that are not necessarily elemental are appropriate for treatment. Current innovations include the use of exclusion and reintroduction diets as a method of maintaining remission in patients. Maintenance of remission rates up of 59% at 2 years have been reported using this approach.

BOWEL REST AS SUPPORTIVE THERAPY

The benefit of bowel rest and parenteral nutrition as supportive therapy in patients with CD has been demonstrated in patients who receive preoperative nutrition support. Prospective randomized-controlled studies have shown that perioperative parenteral nutrition reduces postoperative complications in severely malnourished patients if given for at least 7 to 10 days.[3] Furthermore, retrospective studies have shown fewer postoperative complications, and a decreased length of bowel resection occurs when parenteral nutrition is administered preoperatively in patients with CD.[4] Parenteral nutrition may also be used as supportive therapy in patients with colitis, which has generally been resis-

---

Table 30-1
Indication for Parenteral Nutrition in Crohn's Disease

Gastrointestinal Dysfunction
- Short bowel syndrome
- Severe malabsorption
- High output fistula
- Obstruction and ileus
- Intractable vomiting and diarrhea
- GI bleeding
- Severe colitis
- Bowel ischemia

---

tant to enteral nutrition as primary therapy, in those with severe intestinal dysfunction, and when enteral access is not possible. These conditions are outlined in Table 30-1.

BOWEL REST AS PRIMARY THERAPY

The use of bowel rest with the institution of parenteral nutrition in patients with CD has been addressed and disputed by studies in the past. The consensus by the American Society for Parenteral and Enteral Nutrition (ASPEN) is that parenteral nutrition does not have a primary role as treatment aimed at inducing remission in CD.[5] The use of parenteral nutrition comes with many risks to patients and therefore it is not an appropriate treatment method.

The application of bowel rest with parenteral nutrition as primary therapy in patients with an ECF can develop as a result of CD or as a complication of surgery. Fistula output can be reduced by making a patient NPO (nil per os, "nothing by mouth"), and may help promote fistula closure. Parenteral nutrition is applied concurrently to maintain nutrient, fluid, electrolyte, and acid-base status. Maintaining NPO status for 7 days after the fistula has closed is recommended prior to resuming oral intake. ECF related to surgery have a better response than those as a result of CD itself. Octreotide is sometimes used as an adjunctive medication to promote fistula closing to minimize fluid and electrolyte losses.

SUMMARY

The main goal of nutrition support is to correct the nutritional deficiencies in patients with CD. The enteral route is the preferred method for providing this support. The use of dietary modification and supplementation is the most common approach, especially in patients where nutrient deficiencies are mild to moderate in severity. Enteral nutrition can also be used as primary treatment in patients with active CD. Advantages of this approach include limiting the patient's exposure to immunosuppressive therapy, especially corticosteroids, and correction of nutritional deficiencies. Parenteral nutrition, on the other hand, does not have a primary role in the treatment of patients with CD. The indications for parenteral nutrition in CD are similar to those for patients without IBD. The application of nutrition support, whether it is enteral or parenteral nutrition, requires a great degree of dedication from the clinician and the patient as intolerance and side effects are common and need to be avoided or managed as they arise. Nutritional therapies are an important component of the care of most patients with CD and, when done appropriately, can lead to an improvement in patient care outcomes and quality of life.

References

1. Goh J, O'Morain CA. Review article: nutrition and adult inflammatory bowel disease. *Aliment Pharmacol Ther.* 2003;17(3):307-320.
2. ASPEN Board of Directors. Inflammatory bowel disease: guidelines for the use of parenteral and enteral nution in adult and pediatric patients. *J Parent Enteral Nutr.* 2002;26(1):73SA-74SA.
3. The Veterans Affairs Total Parenteral Nutrition Cooperative Study Group. Perioperative total parenteral nutrition in surgical patients. *NEJM.* 1991;325(8):525-532.
4. Kelly DG. Nutrition in inflammatory bowel disease. *Cur Gastro Rep.* 1999;1(4):324-330.
5. Lashner BA, Evans AA, Hanauer SB. Preoperative total parenteral nutrition for bowel resection in Crohn's disease. *Dig Dis Sci.* 1989;34(5):741-746.

How Do You Treat Microscopic Colitis?

Darrell S. Pardi, MD, FACG, AGAF

The first point to consider in the management of patients with microscopic colitis is to ensure that the diagnosis is correct. In some cases, normal colon biopsies read by an inexperienced pathologist can be misdiagnosed as showing microscopic colitis when normal amounts of inflammatory cells in the lamina propria are misinterpreted as abnormal. The understanding that the primary histologic abnormality in microscopic colitis is intraepithelial lymphocytosis should minimize the risk of this error. Furthermore, even if the diagnosis of microscopic colitis is correct, it should be recognized that there is an increased risk of celiac sprue in these patients.[1] This association should be considered and assessed, particularly for those patients with severe symptoms, significant weight loss or other clues to malabsorption (such as iron deficiency anemia or metabolic bone disease), or lack of response to the usual medications for microscopic colitis. For those patients with concomitant celiac sprue, prompt instruction on a strict gluten-free diet is essential.

Furthermore, the entity of drug-induced microscopic colitis needs to be considered.[2] A thorough review of the patient's medication list, including over-the-counter medications, is essential since several commonly used medications (including non-steroidal anti-inflammatory drugs [NSAIDs], aspirin, proton pump inhibitors [PPI], and others) may cause microscopic colitis.[2] In these cases, discontinuation of the offending agent may lead to the complete resolution of colitis and its symptoms. Finally, other common conditions that may worsen diarrhea (such as lactose intolerance), should be excluded.

Regarding medical therapy of microscopic colitis, several large, open-label case series suggest that nonspecific antidiarrheal medications, including loperamide, diphenoxylate, and bile acid-binding agents such as cholestyramine may be effective in a majority of patients.[1] In my experience, these agents are typically tried empirically by patients and primary care physicians before the patient is referred for a gastroenterology consultation.

For patients not responding to nonspecific therapy, there are several treatment options. Five-aminosalicylates (5-ASAs) may be effective, but only in a minority of patients. For most patients, these agents only lead to a partial response.[1] Therefore, the 2 major treatment options are bismuth subsalicylate or corticosteroids. Corticosteroids were the most effective therapy for microscopic colitis in several large case series. Budesonide appears to be as effective as more systemically active steroids, but with less steroid-related side effects due to limited systemic bioavailability because of high first-pass hepatic metabolism. In fact, budesonide is the best studied medication for microscopic colitis with at least 3 placebo-controlled, randomized, controlled trials in patients with collagenous colitis and another in lymphocytic colitis.[3] Response rates approach 80% to 90%, with response often being noticeable in the first few weeks of treatment.

When I use budesonide therapy, the typical starting dose is 9 mg/day for 6 to 8 weeks. I will typically taper down to 6 mg/day for several days, and then 3 mg/day for several days before stopping. The main drawback to budesonide therapy is a very high rate of recurrent symptoms once the medication is stopped (approximately 60% to 80%). Therefore, patients treated with budesonide often require chronic low-dose therapy or treatment with an immunomodulator such as azathioprine or 6-mercaptopurine (6-MP) for maintenance. If there is an early recurrence after discontinuing therapy, I will then restart budesonide at 3 to 6 mg/day, and taper down to the lowest dose effective for maintaining symptomatic response. In my experience, most patients who require long-term budesonide therapy will respond to 3 mg once a day or even every other day. Only if the patient does not tolerate low dose budesonide or experiences a side effect will I consider immunomodulator therapy.

Bismuth subsalicylate is less well studied than budesonide, but in open label case series and one randomized controlled trial that was never fully published, response rates with bismuth subsalicylate approached those of corticosteroids, with minimal side effects.[1,3] Furthermore, anecdotal experience suggests that maintenance of symptomatic response off of therapy may be higher with bismuth than with budesonide. Therefore, for patients without severe symptoms (eg, dehydration, hypokalemia, or significant fecal incontinence), I will typically begin therapy with bismuth subsalicylate at 3 tablets tid (three times a day) for 8 weeks. If there is significant diarrhea, I will also treat with an antidiarrheal agent such as loperamide at the beginning of bismuth therapy. Loperamide is tapered as the diarrhea responds, and after 8 weeks of therapy, bismuth is discontinued. If there is a prompt recurrence of diarrhea with the discontinuation of therapy, I will either try low-dose bismuth or low-dose budesonide for maintenance. If there is a more prolonged remission followed by recurrence later on, I will try another 6- to 8-week course of bismuth.

The large majority of patients with microscopic colitis will respond to treatment with bismuth or budesonide. In those few who do not, I redouble my efforts to ensure the correct diagnosis and to exclude drug-induced microscopic colitis, concomitant celiac sprue, and other causes of diarrhea. If microscopic colitis remains the only identifiable cause of symptoms, I will consider other treatments, such as mesalamine or cholestyramine, recognizing that the evidence base for these treatments is less than that for bismuth or budesonide. I am also aware of a very small number of patients who were treated with infliximab for refractory microscopic colitis, but a larger experience will be necessary to understand the role of this therapy in the treatment algorithm of microscopic colitis. In our practice, less than 1% of patients with microscopic colitis come to surgery for medically refractory disease. In these rare cases, options include diverting ileostomy (which has been shown to lead to resolution of diarrhea and histologic evidence of collagenous colitis) and proctocolectomy, with or without ileal pouch-anal anastomosis (IPAA).

References

1. Pardi DS. Microscopic colitis: an update. *Inflamm Bowel Dis.* 2004;10(6):860-870.
2. Chande N, McDonald JW, MacDonald JK. Interventions for treating collagenous colitis. *Cochrane Database Syst Rev.* 2006;(4):CD003575.
3. Beaugerie L, Pardi DS. Drug-induced microscopic colitis: proposal for a scoring system and review of the literature. *Aliment Pharmacol Ther.* 2005;22(4):277-284.

SHOULD I DILATE COLONIC STRICTURES IN PATIENTS WITH CROHN'S DISEASE?

Jerome D. Waye, MD, FACG, AGAF, FASGE

The decision whether to dilate a stricture in Crohn's disease (CD) depends on the patient's symptoms.

Tight strictures may present with no symptoms, but with the same narrowed lumen, another patient may complain of postprandial abdominal bloating or distention, or with complete or incomplete intestinal obstruction. In the presence of obstructive symptoms, treatment is indicated.

For each stricture, a determination must be made as to whether it is benign or malignant. Strictures in ulcerative colitis (UC) need to be especially scrutinized to be sure that malignancy is not present, whereas strictures in CD most often are benign. It is safe in CD to downsize the scope or use a gastroscope to intubate strictures without dilation and take surveillance biopsies proximal to the stricture. A gastroscope often can be passed to the cecum after stricture intubation, using techniques of abdominal pressure and straightening.

The most common sites for strictures in CD are in the terminal ileum, at ileocolonic anastomoses, and in the colon (as opposed to the small bowel). In the recent literature concerning treatment, the type of strictures, either anastomotic or primary, were about evenly divided.

If the decision has been made to treat a stricture, only a few choices are available. Unfortunately, strictures commonly recur after surgical resection, and these recurrences may lead to the necessity for repeated surgery. Stents may be useful, but self-expanding metal stents should be avoided in benign strictures. Metal stents should only be used under severe extenuating circumstances since they often migrate and may result in the need for emergency surgery. Polyflex stents (Boston Scientific, Natick, MA) are a variety of self-expanding plastic stents (SEPS) that are increasingly used to treat obstruction in the gastrointestinal (GI) tract. These stents are readily placed and can be removed even after having been in place for several months.[1]

The major method for treating stenoses in CD is endoscopic balloon dilation. This can delay the need for surgery and has a high rate of immediate success. However, recurrence of strictures is common. In general, fibrous strictures respond better to mechanical dilation, whereas inflammatory strictures may not respond as well.[2] Most of the papers that discuss balloon dilation avoid patients whose luminal narrowing is related to active inflammation with ulcerations and obvious signs of a peri-stricture inflammatory response.

Dilation involves elongating and/or rupturing fibrous, collagen-rich tissue, which may provoke further inflammation and fibrosis at that site, ultimately leading to recurrence. This has been the experience with stricture dilation.

The overall success rates for balloon dilation have varied from 51% to 85%, and complication rates from 0 to 15%. There is a wide variation in balloon size, technique of balloon expansion, and time that the balloon is inflated.

Technical success for endoscopic balloon dilation is defined in almost all of the papers as the ability to traverse the stricture post-dilation with a colonoscope. However, the introduction of small-caliber pediatric colonoscopes has impacted on that definition.

TECHNIQUE OF BALLOON DILATION

Gentamicin and a penicillin derivative may be given prior to the procedure. However, this is not a universal practice.[3]

The size of the balloon may vary up to 15 to 20 mm in diameter, and may be held at appropriate pressure for 2 minutes and repeated once or twice. Some keep the balloon inflated for a maximum of 5 minutes.

Should steroids be injected to prevent stricture recurrence? The standard technique is to inject triamcinolone (40 mg/mL in 0.5 to 1.0 mL aliquots) using a flexible needle into the most inflamed and narrowed area of the stricture following dilation. A retrospective data collection[3] reported on the success of steroid injection in 11 strictures in 10 patients. A recurrence rate of strictures was seen in 10% of the steroid group (with one perforation) and 31% in the group without steroids (this was a non-randomized paper with no controls, and the decision as to whether to inject with steroids was strictly up to the endoscopist). An editorial[4] on this report questioned whether injection of long-acting steroids truly decreases clinical recurrence of strictures, and it suggested a randomized study. This editorial also noted that virtually all of the evidence for balloon dilation is uncontrolled, and although immediate success rates vary between 80% to 100%, symptomatic recurrence and need for endoscopic re-intervention is considerable.

A randomized study was recently completed in 13 patients at St. Mark's Hospital (London), and it noted that quadrantic steroid infections following dilation showed a trend for a worse outcome.[5] Van Assche, in another editorial, agrees that, at the present time, intramural steroid injection as an adjuvant strategy should not be considered in clinical practice.[6]

A table of all recent papers is presented. It shows the number of patients, number of dilations performed, the number of perforations (ranging from 0 to 11%), the recurrence rate, and the percentage of these strictures that went on to have surgery (Table 32-1).

Table 32-1
Crohn's Disease Strictures: Results of Balloon Dilation

Reference	# Patients	# Strictures	% Success	% Perfs	% Recurrent	% Surgery
Blomberg	27	137	66%	7%	33%	NR
Breysem	18	18	78%	0%	33%	27%
Junge/Zuchnr	10	11	80%	0%	13%	NR
Couckuyt et al	55	78	62%	11%	62% at 5 years	38% at 5 years
Dear/Hunter	22	71	73%	0%	33%	27%
Thomas-Gibs	59	124	77%	5%	59%	59%
Sabate et al	38	53	84%	3%	36% at 1 year	26% at 1 year
Morini et al	43	45	79%	0%	37%	26%
Brooker et al	14	25	50%	0%	29%	21%
Singh et al	17	29	77%	10%	10%	24%
Ferlitsch et al	46	73	85%	3%	62%	28%
East et al	13	13	75%	0%	50%	NR

Adapted from Ajlouni et al.[7]

Perfs = Perforations
% recurrent = recurrent strictures after dilation
% Surgery = those who subsequently had surgery

CONCLUSION

Stricture dilation can delay or prevent the need for surgery in patients with symptomatic strictures in CD, but asymptomatic strictures do not require therapy. Patients with anastomotic strictures respond better to dilation than spontaneous strictures. The complication is most often perforation, and may occur in a significant number of patients (up to 10% of dilations). Most endoscopists who dilate CD strictures do so only for fibrotic strictures and not for those associated with active inflammation. There are various techniques for balloon dilations, but balloons over 20 mm in size should probably be avoided since the use of smaller caliber balloons may be associated with a lower perforation rate. Steroid injections are not recommended. The advent of Polyflex stents may change the entire approach to fibrotic non-anastomotic strictures in CD, and the future for treatment of strictures using these stents is unknown at the present time.

References

1. Garcia-Cano J. Dilation of benign strictures in the esophagus and colon with polyflex stent: a case series study. *Dig Dis Sci.* 2008;53(2):341-346.
2. Breysem Y, Janssens JF, Coremans G, Vantrappen G, Hendrickx G, Rutgeerts P. Endoscopic balloon dilation of colonic and ileo-colonic Crohn's strictures: long-term results. *Gastrointest Endosc.* 1992;38(2):142-147.
3. Singh VV, Draganov P, Valentine J. Efficacy and safety of endoscopic balloon dilation of symptomatic upper and lower gastrointestinal Crohn's disease strictures. *J Clin Gastroenterol.* 2005;39(4):284-290.
4. Van Assche G. Is endoscopic balloon therapy an effective treatment for patients with Crohn's disease strictures? *Nat Clin Pract Gastroenterol Hepatol.* 2005;2(7):298-299.
5. East JE, Brooker JC, Rutter MD, Saunders BP. A pilot study of intrastricture steroid versus placebo injection after balloon dilatation of Crohn's strictures. *Clin Gastroenterol Hepatol.* 2007;5(9):1065-1069.
6. Van Assche G. Intramural steroid injection and endoscopic dilation for Crohn's disease. *Clin Gastroenterol Hepatol.* 2007;5(9):1027-1028.
7. Ajlouni Y, Iser JH, Gibson PR. Endoscopic balloon dilatation of intestinal strictures in Crohn's disease: safe alternative to surgery. *J Gastroenterol Hepatol.* 2007;22(4):486-490.

Is There a Role For Measuring C-Reactive Protein, Erythrocyte Sedimentation Rate, or Fecal Calprotectin in My Inflammatory Bowel Disease Patients?

Paul Rutgeerts, MD, PhD, FRCP; Gert van Assche, MD, PhD; and Séverine Vermeire, MD, PhD

Biomarkers are used commonly in inflammatory bowel disease (IBD) patients in various clinical settings. They are frequently measured during the work-up of a patient suspected of having IBD, and are used to differentiate IBD from other disorders causing chronic diarrhea, abdominal cramps, bleeding, or mucus discharge. Once the diagnosis of IBD has been established, biomarkers remain part of the follow-up to assess disease activity and to monitor the effect of therapies. At present, there is no single golden marker. Instead, various biomarkers are being used, of which C-reactive protein (CRP) and erythrocyte sedimentation rate (ESR) are probably most widely applied. CRP has many advantages, but its short half-life makes this a particularly good marker to detect and follow up disease activity.[1-3] ESR is the velocity with which erythrocytes migrate through the plasma. Although a good marker of inflammation, ESR has disadvantages over CRP as its value is dependent of physiological conditions such as plasma concentration, number, and size of the erythrocytes. In addition, conditions such as anemia, polycytemia, and thalassemia affect ESR. The half-life of ESR is also much longer compared to CRP, and it may take several days before sedimentation rates become normal. Lastly, ESR is affected by age as levels start to increase over the age of 40 years.[4] Other markers such as white blood cell count, ferritin, and platelet count are also valuable to get a global picture of the disease process and the inflammatory state. More recently, fecal markers have come under scrutiny. These markers hold specific promise in IBD as stools are easily accessible.

A number of neutrophil-derived proteins have been studied, including fecal lactoferrin, lysozyme, elastase, myeloperoxidase, and calprotectin.[5-7] Most of these markers are stable, resistant to degradation, and easy to use, and several commercial assays are available. Calprotectin (S100A8/A9) is a calcium- and zinc-binding protein belonging to the family of the S100 proteins, and it is one of the stool markers that has been investigated most intensively. Calprotectin further represents the majority (60%) of cytosolic proteins in the granulocytes. The presence of calprotectin in the feces can therefore be seen as directly proportional to the homing of neutrophils to the intestine.

In the diagnostic work-up of a patient suspected of having IBD, biomarkers are helpful in prioritizing further examinations, including endoscopy, and/or in the decision to start or intensify treatment. In many older studies, CRP and/or ESR were shown to be the markers of choice to differentiate IBD from functional disorders. More recently, several studies have demonstrated the high accuracy of fecal calprotectin in diagnosing IBD and, more specifically, in the differential diagnosis between irritable bowel syndrome (IBS) and IBD.[8,9] Although calprotectin and lactoferrin are very sensitive markers to detect inflammation in the GI tract, they are not specific for IBD, and increased levels are also found in neoplasia, non-steroidal anti-inflammatory drug (NSAID) abuse, infections, and polyps. In children with abdominal symptoms and diarrhea, a positive test for calprotectin or lactoferrin may prioritize endoscopy. Fecal lactoferrin, a 76 kiloDalton (kDa) iron-binding glycoprotein, is also a major component of the granules of neutrophils. Again, this stool marker was found to be increased in Crohn's disease (CD) and ulcerative colitis (UC) patients compared to IBS or healthy controls.[10] The most recent marker on the list, and also from the S100 family, is fecal S100A12, previously called Calgranulin C or EN-RAGE. Excellent accuracy has been reported for detecting inflammation in IBD patients.[11,12] Most recently, investigators have directly compared the accuracy of serum markers CRP and ESR to fecal markers and have even demonstrated superiority of fecal markers over serum markers for discrimination of IBD from IBS or healthy controls.[12,13]

SEVERITY OF INFLAMMATION

Once the diagnosis of IBD has been established, markers of inflammation should remain part of the follow-up. They not only reflect the patient's general condition and activity of the disease, but they are helpful for evaluation of therapies. Generally speaking, a CRP between 10 to 40 mg/L points toward mild inflammation. Severe active inflammation or bacterial infection will typically generate much higher CRP levels, and very high levels (> 200 to 250 mg/L) should raise the suspicion of complications as an abscess. Although CRP is up-regulated in most inflammatory diseases, there is a remarkable difference in CRP response between CD and UC.[14-17] CD is associated with a strong CRP response, and there is a good correlation (although not 100%) with clinical disease activity, endoscopic inflammation, and histologic inflammation.[17] In contrast, UC only has a modest to absent CRP response. This is important to keep in mind when using CRP in clinical practice. There is no good explanation for this discrepancy, especially since in UC, increased amounts of interleukin (IL) 6, IL-1beta (β), or tumor necrosis factor alpha (TNF-α)—the triggers for CRP production by the hepatocytes—are detected. However, the possibility that serum IL-6 concentrations might not reach the same levels in UC as in CD, and the fact that in UC the inflammation is limited to the mucosa, may be reasons to explain the difference.[18] The fecal markers have also been shown to correlate well with the degree of inflammation on endoscopy.[19]

Markers can be valuable to predict relapse. A French study followed patients with medically induced clinical remission and had biological markers evaluated every 6 weeks.[20] Over time, 38/71 patients (53%) relapsed. Two markers were predictive of relapse: CRP > 20 mg/L and ESR > 15 mm. Based on these 2 markers, the authors derived a predictive score and showed that the relative risk (RR) of short-term relapse for patients with a positive score compared to those with a negative score was 8 (95% confidence interval 2.8 to 22.9). Although this score needs confirmation, it could be a simple and easy tool for physicians in the follow-up of patients in clinical remission.

The most difficult scenario for a clinician is probably when IBD patients present with symptoms mimicking a flare while all inflammatory markers remain normal. In that case, it is difficult to know if symptoms are indeed inflammation-related, or whether they are of functional origin. In an Australian study, approximately 10% of patients had a normal CRP despite having active CD on imaging studies.[21] The patients with low or normal CRP more often had pure ileal disease (95% versus 53%) and less colitis (0% versus 24%). Somewhat different figures were observed in a Belgian study, where 28 consecutive CD patients with active disease (Crohn's Disease Activity Index [CDAI] above 150) but with normal CRP levels underwent full colonoscopy with Crohn's Disease Endoscopy Index of Severity (CDEIS). Intriguingly, almost all of the patients (93%) had endoscopic lesions, although the majority were mild (CDEIS ≤ 6).[22] The authors also examined if other markers of inflammation (fecal calprotectin, blood fibrinogen, acid α-1 glycoprotein, or ESR) would be positive and thus represent "better" indicators of inflammation. The fecal calprotectin levels were mildly increased in most patients, but did not correlate with the endoscopic severity, nor was the endoscopic score of severity associated with any of the other biological markers.

In conclusion, biomarkers of inflammation, measured in the serum or in the stools, are useful and should be part of the work-up of patients suspected for IBD. CRP is the biomarker of choice in the blood at least for CD, but it performs less well in UC. Stool markers are increasingly being promoted as noninvasive markers of inflammation and are particularly interesting in patients presenting with chronic diarrhea given the easy accessibility and their specificity to detect intestinal inflammation. Finally, one must not forget that in the diagnosis of IBD, no marker will replace endoscopy with histopathology, and the diagnosis should still include a combination of clinical symptoms and signs together with an objective measurement of inflammatory lesions showing chronic inflammation with the typical features of CD or colitis (chronic architectural distortion, granulomas, cryptitis, crypt abscesses, etc).

Which test or marker of inflammation to use should be decided individually, taking into account its convenience, cost issues, availability, and accuracy, as well as specific qualities (specificity, correlation with severity of inflammation).

References

1. Ballou SP, Kushner I. C-reactive protein and the acute phase response. *Adv Intern Med.* 1992;37:313-336.
2. Gabay C, Kushner I. Acute-phase proteins and other systemic responses to inflammation. *N Engl J Med.* 1999;340(6):448-454.
3. Pepys MB. C-reactive protein fifty years on. *Lancet.* 1981;1(8221):653-657.
4. Osei-Bimpong A, Meek JH, Lewis SM. ESR or CRP? A comparison of their clinical utility. *Hematology.* 2007;12(4):353-357.

5. Langhorst J, Elsenbruch S, Mueller T, et al. Comparison of 4 neutrophil-derived proteins in feces as indicators of disease activity in ulcerative colitis. *Inflamm Bowel Dis*. 2005;11(12):1085-1091.

6. Lundberg JO, Hellström PM, Fagerhol MK, Weitzberg E, Roseth AG. Technology insight: calprotectin, lactoferrin and nitric oxide as novel markers of inflammatory bowel disease. *Nat Clin Pract Gastroenterol Hepatol*. 2005;2(2):96-102.

7. Sugi K, Saitoh O, Hirata I, Katsu K. Fecal lactoferrin as a marker for disease activity in inflammatory bowel disease: comparison with other neutrophil-derived proteins. *Am J Gastroenterol*. 1996;91(5):927-934.

8. Tibble JA, Sigthorsson G, Foster R, et al. High prevalence of NSAID enteropathy as shown by a simple fecal test. *Gut*. 1999;45(3):362-366.

9. Fagerberg UL, Loof L, Myrdal U, Hansson LO, Finkel Y. Colorectal inflammation is well predicted by fecal calprotectin in children with gastrointestinal symptoms. *J Pediatr Gastroenterol Nutr*. 2005;40(4):450-455.

10. Walker TR, Land ML, Kartashov A, et al. Fecal lactoferrin is a sensitive and specific marker of disease activity in children and young adults with inflammatory bowel disease. *J Pediatr Gastroenterol Nutr*. 2007;44(4):414-422.

11. de Jong NS, Leach ST, Day AS. Fecal S100A12: a novel noninvasive marker in children with Crohn's disease. *Inflamm Bowel Dis*. 2006;12(7):566-572.

12. Kaiser T, Langhorst J, Wittkowski H, et al. Fecal S100A12 as non-invasive marker distinguishing inflammatory bowel disease from irritable bowel syndrome. *Gut*. 2007;56(12):1706-1713.

13. Schoepfer AM, Trummler M, Seeholzer P, Seibold-Schmid B, Seibold F. Discriminating IBD from IBS: comparison of the test performance of fecal markers, blood leukocytes, CRP, and IBD antibodies. *Inflamm Bowel Dis*. 2008;14(1):32-39.

14. Fagan EA, Dyck RF, Maton PN, et al. Serum levels of C-reactive protein in Crohn's disease and ulcerative colitis. *Eur J Clin Invest*. 1982;12(4):351-359.

15. Niederau C, Backmerhoff F, Schumacher B, Niederau C. Inflammatory mediators and acute phase proteins in patients with Crohn's disease and ulcerative colitis. *Hepatogastroenterology*. 1997;44(13):90-107.

16. Saverymuttu SH, Hodgson HJ, Chadwick VS, Pepys MB. Differing acute phase responses in Crohn's disease and ulcerative colitis. *Gut*. 1986;27(7):809-813.

17. Solem CA, Loftus EV Jr, Tremaine WJ, Harmsen WS, Zinsmeister AR, Sandborn WJ. Correlation of C-reactive protein with clinical, endoscopic, histologic, and radiographic activity in inflammatory bowel disease. *Inflamm Bowel Dis*. 2005;11(8):707-712.

18. Gross V, Andus T, Caesar I, Roth M, Scholmerich J. Evidence for continuous stimulation of interleukin-6 production in Crohn's disease. *Gastroenterology*. 1992;102(2):514-519.

19. Røseth AG, Aadland E, Grzyb K. Normalization of fecal calprotectin: a predictor of mucosal healing in patients with inflammatory bowel disease. *Scand J Gastroenterol*. 2004;39(10):1017-1020.

20. Consigny Y, Modigliani R, Colombel JF, Dupas JL, Lémann M, Mary JY, Groupe d'Etudes Thérapeutiques des Affections Inflammatoires Digestives (GETAID). A simple biological score for predicting low risk of short-term relapse in Crohn's disease. *Inflamm Bowel Dis*. 2006;12(7):551-557.

21. Florin TH, Paterson EW, Fowler EV, Radford-Smith GL. Clinically active Crohn's disease in the presence of a low C-reactive protein. *Scand J Gastroenterol*. 2006;41(3):306-311.

22. Denis MA, Reenaers C, Fontaine F, Belaïche J, Louis E. Assessment of endoscopic activity index and biological inflammatory markers in clinically active Crohn's disease with normal C-reactive protein serum level. *Inflamm Bowel Dis*. 2007;13(9):1100-1105.

WHAT IS THE DEFINITION OF CORTICOSTEROID DEPENDENCE? HOW DO I TREAT PATIENTS WITH CORTICOSTEROID-DEPENDENT INFLAMMATORY BOWEL DISEASE?

David Kotlyar, BS; Wojciech Blonski, MD, PhD; and Gary R. Lichtenstein, MD

Since the seminal study by Truelove and Witts in 1955, therapy with corticosteroids has remained a mainstay of treatment for patients with inflammatory bowel disease (IBD).[1] Unfortunately, some patients will either not respond to corticosteroids, or they will become dependent on corticosteroids with immediate symptomatic recurrence if their corticosteroids therapy is stopped or their dosage is lowered. The definition of corticosteroid dependence has varied. However, a recent well-accepted definition is a relapse of IBD-related symptoms either within 30 days after cessation of corticosteroids or during corticosteroid dose reduction, preventing discontinuation of treatment with corticosteroids for greater than 1 year.[2]

The use of corticosteroids for the treatment of patients with active IBD has potential to cause deleterious effects. Their use is associated with both long- and short-term side effects that can be life threatening. Complications with the use of corticosteroids include striae, osteoporosis, osteonecrosis, increased insulin resistance, weight gain, increased risk of coronary artery disease and cerebrovascular disease, and increased susceptibility toward infections.[3] One study from the TREAT (Crohn's Therapy Resource, Evaluation, and Assessment Tool) registry showed that patients on corticosteroids had elevated risks of death with an odds ratio (OR) of 2.10 (CI 1.15-3.83) and of serious infection with an OR of 2.21 (CI 1.46-3.34).[4] A second study also found that patients on corticosteroids had an elevated rate of postoperative infectious complications.[5]

A population-based inception cohort study observed that, among patients with Crohn's disease (CD) or ulcerative colitis (UC) receiving corticosteroids, 84% of them had either complete or partial response, and 16% of them did not respond to treatment over the first 30 days.[1] However, within 1 year of initial use of corticosteroids, 28% of CD patients and 22% of UC patients were corticosteroid-dependent, and 38% of CD patients and 29% of UC patients underwent surgery.[1] A similar study that focused on pediatric patients with UC demonstrated a corticosteroid-dependency rate of 14%, while 29% required surgery even after 1 year of corticosteroids therapy.[6]

In evaluating the clinical course of patients with CD who were treated with corticosteroids, a recent study highlighted that, of 196 patients with CD, 39 (36%) remained corticosteroid-dependent: 24 who had complete response suffered from immediate relapse upon cessation of corticosteroids, and 15 relapsed after a partial response on corticosteroids.[2] There was no association between relapse and the severity of diarrhea, abdominal pain, weight loss, fever, gender, age, or regional involvement of disease.[2]

Patients with corticosteroid-dependent IBD should receive specific medical therapy in an effort to attempt to withdraw corticosteroids while maintaining clinical remission.[7] In patients with corticosteroid-dependent IBD, the most commonly used drugs are immunomodulators such as azathioprine or 6-mercaptopurine (6-MP).[7] Our recommendations, as established in the American Gastroenterological Association (AGA) guidelines, would be to initiate therapy with azathioprine and/or 6-MP therapy once corticosteroid dependency is established.[7] A dosing of 1 to 1.5 mg/kg daily of 6-MP or 2 to 3 mg/kg daily of azathioprine may be helpful in decreasing or eliminating the needed corticosteroids dose.[7]

Concomitant use of mesalamine is not advocated for use in patients with corticosteroid-dependent CD since it is ineffective in improving clinical outcomes, and may on rare occasion have potential interactive side effects such as leukopenia.[6] Prior to using azathioprine or 6-MP, we recommend a complete blood count (CBC), and once antimetabolite therapy is initiated, this should be assessed every 1 to 2 weeks and eventually, no less frequently than every 3 months.[7] Also, we recommend measurement of thiopurine methyltransferase (TPMT) enzyme activity in all patients prior to initiating antimetabolite therapy with either 6-MP or azathioprine in an effort to prevent adverse effects such as severe myelosuppression.[7]

For patients with CD only, methotrexate (MTX) may be given at a dose of 15 or 25 mg SC (subcutaneously) or IM (intramuscularly) weekly.[7] Use of MTX in patients with UC has been ineffective for induction or maintenance of remission. Patients who use MTX must avoid becoming pregnant while on medication since MTX is a recognized teratogen.[3] For those patients who have severely active steroid refractory UC, cyclosporine is also an option (2 to 4 mg/kg daily) but concurrent use of azathioprine or 6-MP therapy is required to maintain remission.[7] For either CD or UC, another option is infliximab, a monoclonal antibody directed against tumor necrosis factor alpha (TNF-α). This agent should initially be administered as induction therapy via an infusion over 2 hours at a dose of 5 mg/kg at weeks zero, 2, and 6, and then subsequently followed by maintenance infusion every 8 weeks.[7] If the symptoms recur sooner, dosing can be given as frequently as every 4 weeks. If symptomatic recurrence is more frequent than every 4 weeks, then dose escalation to 10 mg/kg every 4 to 8 weeks is advocated. Infusions should be done at a specialized center or outpatient facility to optimally manage possible transfusion reactions.[7] Second-generation corticosteroids such as budesonide undergo rapid first-pass metabolism in the liver as well as in erythrocytes, thus lowering the potential for occurrence of systemic side effects. These second-generation corticosteroids have been demonstrated to be as efficacious as first-generation corticosteroids in patients with mild to moderate CD, thus making them attractive efficacious options.[2]

Corticosteroids have wide-ranging potential adverse effects, with the most prominent being the occurrence of serious infectious complications. Their use has been found to significantly increase the rate of patient mortality. In treating patients with IBD, the clinician should strive to avoid long-term use of corticosteroids and appropriately change the medical armamentarium to immunomodulators (including azathioprine, 6-MP, or MTX) and/or infliximab therapy in patients who are found to be steroid-dependent.

References

1. Faubion WA Jr, Loftus EV Jr, Harmsen WS, Zinsmeister AR, Sandborn WJ. The natural history of corticosteroid therapy for inflammatory bowel disease: a population-based study. *Gastroenterology.* 2001;121(2):255-260.
2. Munkholm P, Langholz E, Davidsen M, Binder V. Frequency of glucocorticoid resistance and dependency in Crohn's disease. *Gut.* 1994;35(3):360-362.
3. Yang YX, Lichtenstein GR. Corticosteroids in Crohn's disease. *Am J Gastroenterol.* 2002;97(4):803-823.
4. Lichtenstein GR, Feagan BG, Cohen RD, et al. Serious infections and mortality in association with therapies for Crohn's disease: TREAT registry. *Clin Gastroenterol Hepatol.* 2006;4(5):621-630.
5. Aberra FN, Lewis JD, Hass D, Rombeau JL, Osborne B, Lichtenstein GR. Corticosteroids and immunomodulators: postoperative infectious complication risk in inflammatory bowel disease patients. *Gastroenterology.* 2003;125(2):320-327.
6. Bianchi Porro G, Cassinotti A, Ferrara E, Maconi G, Ardizzone S. Review article: the management of steroid dependency in ulcerative colitis. *Aliment Pharmacol Ther.* 2007;26(6):779-794.
7. Lichtenstein GR, Abreu MT, Cohen R, Tremaine W. American Gastroenterological Association Institute technical review on corticosteroids, immunomodulators, and infliximab in inflammatory bowel disease. *Gastroenterology.* 2006;130(3):935-940.

How Can I Clarify the Diagnosis in My Patient With Indeterminate Colitis?

William J. Tremaine, MD

As clinicians, we assume that a patient with indeterminate colitis (IC) has either Crohn's disease (CD) or ulcerative colitis (UC), and our inability to make a definitive diagnosis is due to the limitations of current medical technology. Distinguishing UC from CD is not crucial for medical therapy because most treatments, including corticosteroids, immune modulators, and infliximab, are effective for both. Whether mesalamine is effective for Crohn's colitis, in addition to UC, is controversial. Resolving the diagnostic uncertainty in a patient with IC becomes critically important if medical therapy fails to control the symptoms and colectomy becomes necessary. If a diagnosis of UC can be made with confidence, then an ileal pouch-anal anastomosis (IPAA) is a good option. In contrast, performing an IPAA in a patient with IC carries an increased risk of postoperative complications, which might require excision of the pouch or a diverting ileostomy. The risk of pouch failure is 6% to 11% for UC, and 10% to 27% for IC according to reports from 2 academic medical centers with a large series and a mean follow-up of about 5 and 10 years, respectively.[1,2] These figures compare to a pouch failure rate of 56% in patients with a preoperative diagnosis of Crohn's colitis and a mean follow-up of about 7 years.[1]

IC is a diagnosis of exclusion, and the tests to exclude UC and CD are imperfect. Colonoscopy is accurate in distinguishing the 2 about 90% of the time, with a diagnosis of IC in the remaining 10%. The most useful time for colonoscopy for the purpose of differentiating CD from UC is prior to starting therapy for symptoms. Once treatment is initiated with 5-aminosalicylates (5-ASAs), corticosteroids, or immunomodulators, the previously confluent mucosal involvement of UC can look patchy or segmental and indistinguishable from CD. Rectal sparing can occur in UC, and even histological rectal sparing has been reported, but most of the time, the rectum is involved histologically, if not endoscopically. Therefore, it is important to biopsy both normal- and abnormal-appearing areas of the colon at colonoscopy to document the histological as well as the endoscopic pattern of involvement. Backwash ileitis, reported in 22% of patients with pancolonic UC, can be difficult to distinguish from Crohn's ileitis. However, backwash ileitis is not a feature of left-sided UC, and the finding of ileitis with a normal right colon is strong evidence for CD.[3]

Upper gastrointestinal (GI) endoscopy was previously touted as a useful way to diagnose CD, particularly in pediatric patients, by identifying focal active chronic gastritis. More recent studies have shown that this type of chronic gastritis is nonspecific, and it can be found in patients with either UC or CD. In addition, nonspecific esophagitis and duodenitis may also be found with either CD or UC.[4]

Wireless capsule endoscopy has held promise for the diagnosis of CD. However, a diagnosis should not be made in a patient with IC based solely on the findings of a few small bowel erosions because the positive predictive value of the technology is too low. Indeed, > 3 small bowel erosions, the criterion that has been used for a diagnosis of CD, may be found in some healthy individuals.[5]

Mucosal biopsies in chronic colitis are usually non-diagnostic. The finding of multiple non-caseating granulomas in the lamina propria in the setting of chronic colitis is convincing for CD, but such granulomas are found in less than 25% of patients with CD.[6] Granulomas may be present at the bases of mucosal crypt abscesses in patients with UC, but an experienced pathologist will easily distinguish these crypt-associated granulomas of UC (composed primarily of foreign body giant cells) from the granulomas of CD, which are primarily aggregates of epithelioid histiocytes.

Anal fissures and superficial fistulas-in-ano can occur in patients with and without inflammatory bowel disease (IBD), so the presence or history of one of these lesions in a patient with IC is not proof that the patient actually has CD. Nevertheless, an anal fissure or a perianal fistula is a tocsin that the patient may actually have CD. If surgery with an IPAA is considered, surgery should be deferred until the perianal disease is healed, and the patient should be informed that the risks of recurrent perianal disease following IPAA are high.

Imaging studies, including computed tomography enterography (CTE), magnetic resonance (MR) enterography, and ultrasonography are useful in diagnosing CD and UC, but they have not been successful in further defining those patients with IC as either CD or UC.

About one-fourth of patients with IC have negative results with 4 of the clinically available serological tests for IBD—anti-*Saccharomyces cerevisiae* antibodies (ACSA), perinuclear antineutrophil cytoplasmic antibodies (pANCA), anti-I2 (an antibody to *Pseudomonas fluorescens*), and anti-OmpC IgA (an antibody to outer membrane porin C of *Escherichia coli*).[7] In one series, patients with IC with one or more positive serologies had a 63% risk of pouchitis compared to a 17% risk among those with negative serological tests for IBD following ileal pouch surgery.[8] This lower figure of 17% in patients with IC and negative serologies is well within the risk of pouchitis for patients with UC, which has been reported as a cumulative risk of up to 50%. With this information, the clinician can counsel the patient with IC and negative serological tests for IBD that his or her chances for a good outcome with pouch surgery are favorable. Whether additional antibody tests such as the anti-flagellin antibody or the anti-synthetic mannoside antibodies will better define IC remains to be seen.

There are no prospective medical treatment trials in patients with IC, probably because the number of patients is small and the diagnosis is difficult to confirm. One retrospective trial using infliximab showed a similar response among those with persistent IC as compared to those patients in whom the diagnosis was later changed to CD.[9]

In conclusion, a patient diagnosed with IC should be informed of the uncertainties of both the diagnosis and the outcomes of potential treatments, particularly for colectomy and IPAA. If serological tests for IBD are negative, a patient with IC is likely to have a good outcome with pouch-anal surgery. Patients with one or more positive serological tests for IBD are likely to have more complications with an IPAA as compared to patients with UC, but the surgery is still a reasonable option despite the increased risks.

References

1. Brown CJ, Maclean AR, Cohen Z, Macrae HM, O'Connor BI, McLeod RS. Crohn's disease and indeterminate colitis and the ileal pouch-anal anastomosis: outcomes and patterns of failure. *Dis Colon Rectum.* 2005;48(8):1542-1549.
2. Yu CS, Pemberton JH, Larson D. Ileal pouch-anal anastomosis in patients with indeterminate colitis: long-term results. *Dis Colon Rectum.* 2000;43(11):1487-1496.
3. Heuschen UA, Hinz U, Allemeyer EH, et al. Backwash ileitis is strongly associated with colorectal carcinoma in ulcerative colitis. *Gastroenterology.* 2001;120(4):841-847.
4. Bousvaros A, Antonioli DA, Colletti RB, et al. Differentiating ulcerative colitis from Crohn disease in children and young adults: report of a working group of the North American Society for Pediatric Gastroenterology, Hepatology, and Nutrition and the Crohn's and Colitis Foundation of America. *J Pediatr Gastroenterol Nutr.* 2007;44(5):653-674.
5. Goldstein JL, Eisen GM, Lewis B, Gralnek IM, Zlotnick S, Fort JG. Video capsule endoscopy to prospectively assess small bowel injury with celecoxib, naproxen plus omeprazole, and placebo. *Clin Gastroenterol Hepatol.* 2005;3(2):133-141.
6. Freeman HJ. Granuloma-positive Crohn's disease. *Can J Gastroenterol.* 2007;21(9):583-587.
7. Joossens S, Colombel JF, Landers C, et al. Anti-outer membrane of porin C and anti-I2 antibodies in indeterminate colitis. *Gut.* 2006;55(11):1667-1669.
8. Hui T, Landers C, Vasiliaukas E, et al. Serologic responses in indeterminate colitis patients before ileal pouch-anal anastomosis may determine those at risk for continuous pouch inflammation. *Dis Colon Rectum.* 2005;48(6):1254-1262.
9. Papadakis KA, Treyzon L, Abreu MT, Fleshnew PR, Targan SR, Vasiliauskas EA. Infliximab in the treatment of medically refractory indeterminate colitis. *Aliment Pharmacol Ther.* 2003;18(7):741-747.

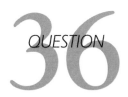

How Should I Treat My Crohn's Patient Postoperatively?

Russell D. Cohen, MD, FACG, AGAF

Crohn's disease (CD) is a chronic recurrent disease that often recurs after surgery. As the location of recurrence is typically at the surgical anastomosis, it has been very easy to study Crohn's recurrence patterns as well as agents to help prevent this recurrence. Roughly one-half to three-quarters of patients who have one Crohn's surgery will have another in their lifetime, so there has been much interest in trying to decrease recurrence rates.

When asking yourself whether you should put a patient on postoperative prophylactic therapy, consider the following:

Is all of the active disease resected? If the patient still has active disease or even evidence of quiescent disease elsewhere in the luminal bowel, then it is advisable to keep him or her on an effective medical therapy. What this therapy is will depend upon the patient's previous experience with medications. However, in the case of patients who have had a "curative" resection of all known active luminal disease, there are a few issues to consider when deciding whether to start someone on postoperative therapy, and how to choose the most appropriate therapy.

The first issue is, "What is the patient's risk of having an early recurrence of CD?" Risk factors for early recurrence of disease include cigarette smoking, penetrating disease (patients who have had internal fistulas, abscesses, or other evidence of penetration through the wall of the bowel), early recurrence since a previous surgery, multiple surgeries, or perhaps a young age at the time of the first surgery. Also, if patients have "burned through" effective medications, one may suspect they have a more aggressive disease and would need to be treated postoperatively. However, be aware that many patients who are first diagnosed with CD as an adult have had years of silent disease with stricturing and subsequent obstruction. They are started on therapies after "the horse is out of the barn," have fibrostenotic strictures, and are already on their way to surgery. The fact that medical therapy was ineffective in preventing surgery does not mean that these patients failed the therapy. Their disease process was too far along for the medical therapy to work.

Another question I ask patients is, "What are your family planning intentions after surgery?" This is particularly an issue for women who may desire a pregnancy after they recover from their surgery. While it is commonly believed that most of the agents that we use are relatively safe for pregnancy, with the notable exception of methotrexate (MTX), there is still much debate about this issue, and one may shy away from immunomodulators for patients in whom a pregnancy is planned soon after recovery.

Once you determine that you are going to discuss postoperative prophylaxis with the patient, the next question is, "What medical options are available, and what is the evidence that they work?" (Table 36-1). The easy agent to prescribe is mesalamine. Mesalamine is a safe therapy, but unfortunately, it has only modest (if any) efficacy in preventing postoperative recurrence, and, historically, it required multiple pills dosed multiple times a day. However, the recent introduction of Lialda (Shire, Wayne, PA) into the marketplace may change that last point. There has been mixed data about whether these agents are effective in preventing postoperative recurrence.[1] Most of the studies that have shown a benefit seem to imply it is limited to ileal disease with doses of mesalamine 2.4 g or higher. When using these agents, if the patient had an ileal resection, I prefer to use Pentasa, as I do not need to rely on a particular intestinal pH for release, as would be the case with Asacol (Proctor & Gamble, Cincinnati, OH) or Lialda. The azo-bond drugs only work in the colon, and if the anastomosis is at the small bowel, then those would not be an appropriate choice, either. I usually dose 3 g or greater, split twice a day (bid).

There has been much interest in using antibiotics in postoperative prevention, as a randomized placebo-controlled trial showed that metronidazole (at 20 mg/kg for 3 months) prevented recurrence of disease.[2] Similar results were shown for ornidazole therapy for 12 months. Unfortunately, both agents were too toxic to continue long-term, and their beneficial effects waned after the medications were stopped. I have used other antibiotics in an uncontrolled fashion such as ciprofloxacin and rifaximin. Hopefully there will be future studies evaluating their efficacy.

The best data so far has been for azathioprine or 6-mercaptopurine (6-MP), even though they have only been well studied in 1 or 2 trials. Even low-dose 6-MP (at 50 mg) has been shown to have a benefit versus placebo in preventing postoperative recurrence, and, nowadays, people often use higher doses of azathioprine or 6-MP (Figure 36-1).[3] Dosing parameters would be similar to that used in patients with active disease, although it may be safer to initially use slightly lower doses and then evaluate how the patient is progressing, as detailed below. There is not enough information on MTX to confirm its efficacy, so I use it in select patients who need a therapy more potent than mesalamine, and who cannot receive the other immunomodulators.

What about other agents that we use in patients with CD? Budesonide has been an effective agent in the treatment of CD; unfortunately, there was no benefit of budesonide versus placebo in preventing a Crohn's relapse. While much attention has been given to the promise of probiotics changing the natural course of CD, there have been no positive placebo-controlled trials to date for postoperative prevention.

While we are still waiting for the publication of adequate placebo-controlled trials with either infliximab or adalimumab in preventing postoperative recurrence, their efficacy in treating active disease and maintaining remission has led me and others to use these agents as postoperative prophylaxis in certain patient groups. One group is the patients who have failed azathioprine, 6-MP, or MTX that had been started immediately after their

Table 36-1

Therapies Tested in Postoperative Prophylaxis for Crohn's Disease

Therapy	Postoperative Prophylaxis Efficacy
Mesalamine	+
Antibiotics (select)	++
Azathioprine/6-mercaptopurine	+++
Methotrexate	?
Budesonide	−
Probiotics	−
Infliximab/adalimumab	?

−	not effective
?	not known if effective
+	mixed data supportive of use
++	data supportive of use; modest efficacy
+++	data supportive of use; good efficacy

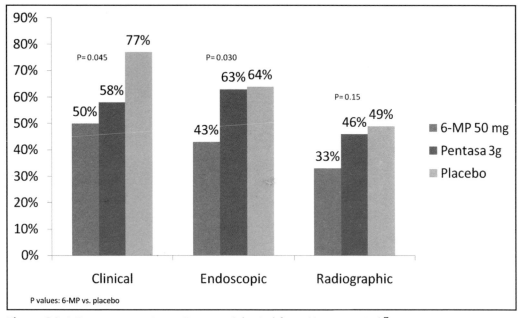

Figure 36-1. Recurrence rates at 2 years. Adapted from Hanauer et al.[7]

previous surgery, and yet they still suffered a disease recurrence. Other groups are those patients who have had multiple surgeries, those with a short bowel or who will have a short bowel after their next surgery, or those who have an allergy, intolerance, or contraindication to other therapies.

One way to guide therapy might be to do a colonoscopy 6 to 12 months following a surgical resection, and then see if the patient has active inflammation. The suggestion is that patients who have 5 or more mucosal lesions on the ileal side after an ileocolonic resection within this time period have more active disease and might prompt you to either increase your therapy to a more effective agent or to just start postoperative therapy as well.[4] The role of capsule endoscopy in monitoring patient recurrence has not yet been established. Since most of the patients' anastomoses are easily reachable by a colonoscope, it is the preferred method at this time. For patients who have surgical anastomoses that are not easily amenable to endoscopic evaluation, a capsule endoscopy may be a good choice. However, in any patient with CD, it is wise to first do a dissolvable patency capsule test to make sure that the capsule endoscope does not get stuck.

Patients who are on effective therapy with any of the agents mentioned above postoperatively and are doing well should be maintained on these therapies unless safety issues arise. Hopefully, more agents will be available in the future and better studies can be conducted to determine efficacy in this condition.

References

1. Camma C, Giunta M, Rosselli M, Cottone M. Mesalamine in the maintenance treatment of Crohn's disease: a meta-analysis adjusted for confounding variables. *Gastroenterology.* 1997;113(5):1465-1473.
2. Rutgeerts P, Hiele M, Geboes K, et al. Controlled trial of metronidazole treatment for prevention of Crohn's recurrence after ileal resection. *Gastroenterology.* 1995;108(6):1617-1621.
3. Hanauer SB, Korelitz BI, Rutgeerts P, et al. Postoperative maintenance of Crohn's disease remission with 6-mercaptopurine, mesalamine, or placebo: a 2-year trial. *Gastroenterology.* 2004;127(3):723-729.
4. Rutgeerts P, Geboes K, Vantrappen G, Beyls J, Kerremans R, Hiele M. Predictability of the postoperative course of Crohn's disease. *Gastroenterology.* 1990;99(4):956-963.

37

IS IT SAFE AND EFFECTIVE TO VACCINATE MY PATIENT WITH INFLAMMATORY BOWEL DISEASE?

Carmen Cuffari, MD

The treatment paradigms in patients with inflammatory bowel disease (IBD) have changed over the last several years. Gastroenterologists have adopted a more aggressive approach to therapy with the early institution of immunosuppressive agents in the management of moderate to severe disease.[1] The balance between immunosuppression and drug toxicity, namely leukopenia, has always been a subject of debate and controversy.[2] Therefore, it would seem reasonable that, whenever possible, infection should be prevented with available vaccines.

In pediatrics, IBD is less common under the age of 5 years.[3] Most patients are diagnosed during their pre-adolescent and adolescent years and, as a result, they have received the full complement of childhood vaccinations.[4] For the very young child with IBD, physicians may worry that the immune response may not be adequate due to the severity of the disease or due to the immunosuppressive medications the patient may be receiving. Often, these children are neglected when it comes to immunization, as has been shown in children with chronic liver disease awaiting liver transplantation.[5] In comparison, older children may have their booster shots and protective vaccinations against influenza, meningococcal, and pneumococcal infections neglected as a consequence to similar concerns.[5] This may also hold true for children with severe IBD on aggressive immunosuppressive therapy, including high dosage (2 mg/kg/day) corticosteroids.[6]

IMMUNE RESPONSE IN IBD

The effectiveness of vaccinations in patients with IBD depend on the patient's innate immune response and the compromising effects of immunosuppressive drugs on that response to infectious pathogens.

In general, patients with IBD have normal serum gamma globulin levels and a number of circulating antibodies to enteric microorganisms, thereby reflecting a primed and robust humoral immunity. These antibodies are produced on intestinal exposure to normal commensual bacteria. An excellent example is anti-CBir1 (flagellin) antibody. The CBir1 flagellin has been shown to elicit a strong CD4 T-cell lymphocyte response in the CRH/HeJBir colitic mouse, and can induce colitis when these activated lymphocytes are transferred to severe combined immunodeficiency (SCID) mice. Flagellin has been defined as a ligand to toll-like receptor 5 (TLR5), the start of which culminates in the activation of nuclear factor kappa-light-chain-enhancer of activated B cells (NF-κB).[7] The induction of colitis on exposure to this antigen is unique among all of the other bacterial antigens listed above where an antibody response has been associated with intestinal disease. Although these antibodies are non-pathogenic, they are specific to patients with Crohn's disease (CD) and may reflect a dysregulated immune inflammatory response to intestinal bacterial antigens.

In comparison, cell-mediated immunity would also seem enhanced in patients with IBD. While the proportions of T and B lymphocytes are similar to those observed in healthy intestinal mucosa, its response to intestinal and environmental stimuli would seem to be also dysregulated. Indeed, patients with CD manifest an exaggerated T helper type 1 (TH1) response, while patients with ulcerative colitis (UC) manifest an inappropriate TH2 response.[8] Although these lymphocytes are quantitatively normal, their response to environmental and bacterial stimuli is not only exaggerated, but it is also resistant to apoptosis. The implication on a patient's ability to mount an effective immune response to vaccination in IBD is unknown.

Several studies have reported on the immune response to vaccination in a number of chronic diseases, including lupus and rheumatoid arthritis (RA). The general consensus is that these patients make adequate antibodies in response to conventional vaccinations, and are not predisposed to an increased risk for disease activation. Although the immunopathogenesis of these chronic systemic disorders is very different to that in patients with IBD, a certain consensus could generally be reached based on this clinical experience until an evidenced-based approach is provided to physicians and surgeons caring for patients with UC and CD (Table 37-1).[9]

IMMUNOSUPPRESSANTS

The effects of corticosteroids on the elderly are well understood. These patients are particularly susceptible to opportunistic infections, as well as the resurgence of herpetic and mycobacterial infections. In children, a safe dose and duration of corticosteroid therapy has yet to be defined, especially among those children scheduled to receive live-virus vaccines. Nevertheless, several guidelines have been adopted by the American Academy of Pediatrics (AAP) (see Table 37-1).[10]

Six-mercaptopurine (6-MP) and its parent compound, azathioprine, have proven efficacy in the treatment of steroid-dependent IBD. They act by interfering with protein synthesis and nucleic acid metabolism in the sequence that follows antigen stimulation, as well as by their direct cytotoxic effects on lymphoid cells.[11] Methotrexate (MTX) is a folic acid antagonist that affects thymidine synthesis and DNA replication. It has been adopted in selected patients with steroid- and azathioprine-resistant CD.[12] Cyclosporine is a peptide that blocks interleukin 2 (IL-2) production by TH cells inhibiting lymphocyte proliferation and lymphokine response to antigen exposure.[13] All 3 have profound effects on the immune system, with cyclosporine being perhaps the more potent immunosup-

Table 37-1

General Recommendations for Immunization of Patients with IBD[9]

- Standard immunization schedules for children and adults should be generally adhered to.
- At diagnosis, all patients with incomplete series should commence catch-up vaccination.
- Adults who cannot provide a clear history of chickenpox should have serologic testing for varicella. Non-immune individuals should receive varicella vaccine. Children who are not immune by vaccination or acquired immunity through infection should receive varicella vaccine.
- Live bacterial or viral vaccines should be avoided in immunocompromised children and adults with IBD. This includes:
  - Treatment with glucocorticoids (> prednisone 20 mg/d equivalent, or 2 mg/kg/d if less than 10 kg, for 2 weeks or more, and within 3 months of stopping)
  - Treatment with effective doses of 6-MP/azathioprine* and within 3 months of stopping
  - Treatment with methotrexate* and within 3 months of stopping
  - Treatment with infliximab* and within 3 months of stopping.
  - Significant protein-calorie malnutrition.

*effect on safety not established

pressive agent. All of these drugs will, to a greater or lesser extent, affect the natural immune response to immunization. It is assumed that patients on immunosuppressants can be safely given denatured protein, carbohydrates, and killed virus vaccines. However, there has been an ongoing concern as to whether seroconversion with effective and long-lasting protective antibody titres can be achieved. Although the AAP has recommended the continued use of a killed virus in immunosuppressed patients, well-designed studies of vaccine safety and efficacy in patients with IBD have yet to be performed. However, a number of conventional and experimental live vaccines have not been recommended in immunocompromised patients (Table 37-2).[9] It would behoove clinicians to include patients with either CD or UC due to the absence of controlled studies.

Live Virus Vaccines

In general, immunocompromised patients are not given live virus vaccines on the concern of developing a vaccine-associated disease. However, most of the concern with live virus vaccines is in patients with HIV or post-transplantation.[14] In IBD, many clinicians would consider high dose (> 20 mg/day) prednisone therapy a contraindication in the use of live virus vaccines. Fortunately, most patients with steroid-dependent or refractory IBD respond well to immunosuppressive agents and are effectively weaned off of corticosteroids.

The severity of measles is enhanced in the immunosuppressed patient. Although there have been anecdotal reports of severe complications post-measles virus infection, most patients have benefited from immunization without a complication. The same would

Table 37-2

Vaccines Contraindicated in Immune Compromised Patients with IBD*[9,10]

Vaccine	Type
Anthrax Vaccine	Absorbed
BCG	Live
Measles Virus Vaccine	Live
Measles, Mumps, and Rubella Virus Vaccine	Live
Mumps Virus Vaccine	Live
Rubella Virus Vaccine	Live
Smallpox (vaccinia) Vaccine	Live
Typhoid Vaccine TY21a	Live, Oral
Varicella Virus Vaccine	Live
Yellow Fever Vaccine	Live
Adenovirus type 4 and 7	Oral, Live
Cholera, attenuated, Vibiro cholera strain CVD 103-HgR	Oral, Live

*high dose (> 20 mg/day) prednisone equivalent for 2 weeks or more, and within 3 months of stopping; significant protein calorie malnutrition.

hold true for the mumps and rubella vaccines. In transplantation, the use of the measles, mumps, and rubella (MMR) vaccines is considered unsafe post-transplant.[15] The same does not hold true in IBD unless the patient is highly immunosuppressed with cyclosporine therapy. In patients with leukemia on long-term 6-MP therapy, the varicella vaccine was well tolerated in most patients, and would also apply in patients with IBD.[16] In these patients, problems with seroconversion were managed with repeat vaccinations. The general consensus for the polio vaccine is to use the inactivated polio vaccine (see Table 37-2).[9] This also applies for unaffected siblings and household contact of patients with IBD that may shed the virus if given the oral vaccine.

INACTIVATED VACCINES

Inactivated vaccines are well tolerated by most immunosuppressed patients. The problems are associated with the ability of patients to seroconvert and maintain immuno-protective antibody titres. This issue has been raised in patients post-transplantation who have received either the pneumococcal or meningococcal vaccine. The general consensus is that these infectious agents pose a serious threat in both pediatric and adult immuno-suppressed patients, and that all patients should be immunized. The concern regarding the adequacy of seroconversion and the maintenance of protective antibody titres can be managed clinically by monitoring serum antibody levels.

In summary, much remains unknown on the safety and efficacy of conventional vaccinations among adults and patients with IBD, especially with live vaccines. Until those pivotal studies are performed, patients with IBD should not deviate from the recommended immunization schedules with close attention to avoiding the use of live vaccines among significantly immunocompromised individuals. The future availability of surrogate immune markers of adequate immune response to conventional vaccinations may also prove helpful in guiding immunization practices in patients with CD and UC.

References

1. Sandborn WJ. Current directions in IBD therapy: what goals are feasible with biological modifiers. *Gastroenterology.* 2008;135(5):1442-1447.
2. Colonna T, Korelitz BI. The role of leukopenia in 6-mercaptopurine-induced remission of refractory Crohn's disease. *Am J Gastroenterol.* 1993;89(3):362-366.
3. Cuffari C, Darbari A. Inflammatory bowel disease in the pediatric and adolescent patient. *Gastroenterol Clin North Am.* 2002;31(1):275-291.
4. American Academy of Pediatrics. Immunization in special circumstances. In: Pickering L, ed. *2000 Red Book: Report of the Committee on Infectious Diseases.* Elk Grove Village, IL: American Academy of Pediatrics; 2000:54-79.
5. Thall TV, Rosh JR, Schwersenz AH, et al. Primary immunization status in infants referred for liver transplantation. *Transplant Proc.* 1994;26(1):191-195.
6. Cuffari C. Inflammatory bowel disease in children: a pediatrician's perspective. *Minerva Pediatr.* 2006;58(2):139-157.
7. Shen C, Landers CJ, Derkowski C, Elson CO, Targan SR. Enhanced CBir1-specific innate adaptive immune responses in Crohn's disease. *Inflamm Bowel Dis.* 2008;14(12):1641-1651.
8. Latinne D, Fiasse R. New insights into the cellular immunology of the intestine in relation to the pathophysiology of inflammatory bowel diseases. *Acta Gastroenterol Belg.* 2006(4);69:393-405.
9. Sands BE, Cuffari C, Katz J, et al. Guidelines for immunization in patients with inflammatory bowel disease. *Inflamm Bowel Dis.* 2004;10(5):677-692.
10. Casswall TH, Fischler B. Vaccination of the immunocompromised child. *Expert Rev Vaccines.* 2005;4(5):725-738.
11. Fairchild CR, Maybaum J, Kennedy KA. Concurrent unilateral chromatid damage and DNA strand breaks in response to 6-thioguanine treatment. *Biochem Pharmacol.* 1986;35(20):3533-3541.
12. Tian H, Cronstein BN. Understanding the mechanisms of action of methotrexate: implications for the treatment of rheumatoid arthritis. *Bull NYU Hosp Jt Dis.* 2007;65(3):168-173.
13. Hamawy MM. Molecular actions of calcineurin inhibitors. *Drug News Perspect.* 2003;16(5):277-282.
14. Durando P, Fenoglio D, Boschini A, et al. Safety and immunogenicity of two influenza virus subunit vaccines, with or without MF59 adjuvant, administered to human immunodeficiency virus type 1-seropositive and seronegative adults. *Clin Vaccine Immunol.* 2008;15(2):253-259.
15. Danerseau AM, Robinson JL. Efficacy and safety of measles, mumps, rubella and varicella live viral vaccines in transplant recipients receiving immunosuppressive drugs. *World J Pediatr.* 2008;4(4):254-258.
16. LaRussa P, Steinberg S, Gershon AA. Varicella vaccine for immunocompromised children: results of collaborative studies in the United States and Canada. *J Infect Dis.* 1996;174(suppl 3):S320-S323.

What Is the Risk of Developing Lymphoma in My Patients With Crohn's Disease, and Do the Immunomodulators and Biologic Agents Increase the Risk?

James D. Lewis, MD, MSCE, AGAF

The fear of medication-induced cancer is among the leading reasons for patients electing not to pursue therapy with the immunomodulators azathioprine or 6-mercaptopurine (6-MP) and anti-tumor necrosis factor (TNF). This chapter will review the data that support or refute the hypothesis that the risk of lymphoma is augmented by therapy with these medications.

To understand this question, it is necessary to first ask whether patients with Crohn's disease (CD) have an increased risk of lymphoma at baseline. The hypothesis that CD would increase the risk of lymphoma draws on similar observations among patients with other immune-mediated diseases, particularly rheumatoid arthritis (RA). Patients with RA have an increased risk of lymphoma that appears to be independent of immunomodulator or anti-TNF therapy and is positively associated with the severity of the RA. However, data to support such an association among patients with CD are generally lacking. While a few studies have documented an increased risk of lymphoma in patients with CD, these were generally small single-center studies. Such studies are potentially biased for a number of reasons.

One source of bias results from including patients whose observation prompts the completion of a study. If a clinician notices a few patients with lymphoma and is therefore prompted to conduct a study on this question, inclusion of the patients that prompted the study will bias the study in favor of a positive finding. Note that clinicians who have not seen a few patients with lymphoma are far less likely to undertake such a study in their own data. As such, small studies that do not show an increased risk are not only less likely to be published, but are probably less likely to even be completed. Another potential bias from single-center studies relates to the fact that clinical centers where research is conducted are more likely to be referral centers for multiple conditions. If a study is completed at a referral center for both CD and lymphoma, there is potential for bias toward a positive study.

In contrast to the small studies addressing the question of CD and lymphoma, most large population-based or population-representative studies have not demonstrated an increased risk of lymphoma among patients with CD compared to the general population. This suggests that, overall, there is no increased risk of lymphoma when patients with CD are viewed as a whole. However, this does not rule out the possibility that patients with the most severe CD could still have a small increased risk of lymphoma. In fact, this is another reason why small referral center studies could show an association when large population-based studies do not. The limited available data from the pre-infliximab era do not suggest this to be the case, but the data are too scant to draw firm conclusions.

Most of the data on the association of medical therapies for CD and the risk of lymphoma come from observational studies, not randomized, controlled trials. Because of this, the issue of whether patients with the most severe CD are at an increased risk of lymphoma is critical to interpreting the data on the association of medical therapies. If the patients with the most severe CD are also the patients who are most likely to be treated with immunomodulators and anti-TNF therapies, an observed association between these therapies and an increased risk of lymphoma could be an artifact of the disease severity. This is referred to as confounding by indication and must be considered when interpreting the results of the observational studies.

Kandiel and colleagues conducted a meta-analysis specifically examining the question of whether patients with inflammatory bowel disease (IBD) who are treated with azathioprine or 6-MP are at an increased risk of lymphoma.[1] This meta-analysis demonstrated an approximately 4-fold increased risk of lymphoma among the patients treated with azathioprine or 6-MP, regardless of whether the control population was the general population or patients with CD who were not treated with these medications. As the studies were conducted, it was not possible to distinguish whether some or all of this increased risk of lymphoma was attributable to the more severe underlying disease. To the extent that this was the case, the increased relative risk (RR) of lymphoma associated with the medical therapy is likely less than that observed within the meta-analysis.

There are several additional key limitations of the Kandiel meta-analysis. First, the studies included in the meta-analysis covered a broad range of time periods, during most of which the doses of azathioprine and 6-MP used were less than that employed in the treatment of CD today. Thus, if the RR of lymphoma is related to the dose of azathioprine or 6-MP, the meta-analysis could have underestimated the RR. Likewise, all of the studies included in the meta-analysis assumed that the RR remained constant, even after the medication was discontinued. If in fact the RR is lower after the medication is discontinued, the meta-analysis may have underestimated the RR during the period in which the patient was actually taking the medication, or shortly thereafter.

The question of whether anti-TNF drugs increase the risk of lymphoma is complicated by several factors. Most importantly, many patients treated with these medications are already at an increased risk of lymphoma, either due to their underlying disease (eg, RA) or as a result of concomitant therapies (eg, azathioprine or 6-MP). Some observational studies have not suggested a further increase in the risk of lymphoma among patients treated with infliximab or adalimumab for CD.[2] Similarly, some large observational studies of patients with RA have not demonstrated an increased risk of lymphoma, although other studies have suggested such an association.[3,4] These observational data must be weighed against the results of a meta-analysis of randomized, placebo-controlled trials of these 2 medications for RA.[5] This meta-analysis demonstrated a higher rate of malignancy (not just lymphoma) among patients treated with anti-TNF drugs compared to placebo, despite the relatively short duration of the studies. Although a lymphoma-specific analysis was not completed, there were 4 cases of lymphoma observed among the patients treated with anti-TNF therapy and none among patients treated with placebo.

The results of this meta-analysis are compelling since the placebo-controlled randomized trials eliminate concern over confounding by indication, and presumably, randomization resulted in balance between the study groups in terms of the use of other medications that could increase the risk of lymphoma. However, the findings are generally inconsistent with our model of cancer development, which typically assumes that several years to even decades are required for cancer to develop. These results, though, could be consistent with an unmasking of preexisting cancers. Of note, lymphomas can behave differently than most solid tumors, presenting rapidly in the setting of severe immunosuppression (eg, AIDS or post-transplant lymphoproliferative disease). As such, the observation of an excess of lymphomas in the placebo-controlled clinical trials is biologically plausible.

Most recently, reports of hepatosplenic T-cell lymphoma (HSTCL) among young patients treated with infliximab has further fueled the debate over whether anti-TNF therapies increase the risk of lymphoma. This rare and frequently lethal form of lymphoma has previously been reported in the setting of immunosuppression. It is notable that nearly all of the reported cases among patients treated with infliximab have occurred in patients receiving concomitant immunomodulators. Many cases have also been reported with corticosteroids as adjunct therapy. Thus, it is possible that these lymphomas have resulted from substantial immunosuppression created by the combination of multiple medications.

Taken together, the available data suggest that patients with CD do not have an increased risk of lymphoma in the absence of medical therapy. Whether severe CD is associated with an increased risk of lymphoma, as has been observed in RA, remains to be answered. Assuming that severe CD does not increase the risk of lymphoma, the use of azathioprine or 6-MP appears to increase the risk of lymphoma approximately 3- to 4-fold above the risk in the general population. Depending on the patient's age, this translates to one additional lymphoma in approximately 400 to 4000 treated patients per year of follow-up.[1] Whether the risk of lymphoma returns to baseline after the medication is discontinued is unknown, but one would expect that the risk is at least lower than when associated with active therapy since at least some lymphomas observed with these medications are due to immunosuppression. Whether treatment with infliximab and adalimumab also increase the risk of lymphoma is the least clear. The cluster of patients with the rare HSTCL and the findings of the meta-analysis of clinical trials suggest that at least the combination of anti-TNF therapies with other immunosuppressants may predispose to certain types of lymphoma, and that these drugs may unmask preexisting tumors.

Lastly, one must ask whether the risks of such therapies outweigh the benefits. Although this question must be answered on a patient-by-patient basis, the available evidence suggests that the risk of lymphoma attributable to azathioprine or 6-MP does not outweigh the potential benefits for most patients.[6] Assuming that the RR of lymphoma among patients treated with anti-TNF therapies is likely as low or lower than that observed with azathioprine or 6-MP, it is logical to conclude that the benefits of anti-TNF therapy would also outweigh the risk of lymphoma. Although definitive data are lacking, a logical hypothesis is that the risk of lymphoma may be reduced by minimizing the number of immunosuppressant medications prescribed, thus supporting a philosophy of discontinuing ineffective therapies. Whether long-term Crohn's-specific outcomes are better with an anti-TNF drug combined with an immunomodulator than with anti-TNF therapy alone remains to be determined, but this would need to be considered in the decision to discontinue immunomodulators in patients treated with anti-TNF therapies.

References

1. Kandiel A, Fraser AG, Korelitz BI, Brensinger C, Lewis JD. Increased risk of lymphoma among inflammatory bowel disease patients treated with azathioprine and 6-mercaptopurine. *Gut*. 2005;54(8):1121-1125.
2. Biancone L, Orlando A, Kohn A, et al. Infliximab and newly diagnosed neoplasia in Crohn's disease: a multi-centre matched pair study. *Gut*. 2006;55(2):228-233.
3. Geborek P, Bladstrom A, Turesson C, et al. Tumour necrosis factor blockers do not increase overall tumour risk in patients with rheumatoid arthritis, but may be associated with an increased risk of lymphomas. *Annals of the Rheumatic Diseases*. 2005;64(5):699-703.
4. Wolfe F, Michaud K. The effect of methotrexate and anti-tumor necrosis factor therapy on the risk of lymphoma in rheumatoid arthritis in 19,562 patients during 89,710 person-years of observation. *Arthritis & Rheumatism*. 2007;56(5):1433-1439.
5. Bongartz T, Sutton AJ, Sweeting MJ, Buchan I, Matteson EL, Montori V. Anti-TNF antibody therapy in rheumatoid arthritis and the risk of serious infections and malignancies: systematic review and meta-analysis of rare harmful effects in randomized controlled trials. *JAMA*. 2006;295(19):2275-2285.
6. Lewis JD, Schwartz S, Lichtenstein G. Azathioprine for maintenance of remission in Crohn's disease: benefits outweigh the risk of lymphoma. *Gastroenterology*. 2000;118(6):1018-1024.

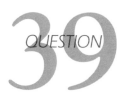

HOW DO YOU DOSE 5-AMINOSALICYLIC ACIDS? WHEN DO YOU USE TOPICAL THERAPY? HOW DO YOU MONITOR DURING THERAPY?

Russell D. Cohen, MD, FACG, AGAF

When I treat patients with Crohn's disease (CD) or ulcerative colitis (UC) and am planning to use a 5-aminosalicylic acid (5-ASA) agent, I consider the following issues:

The first is, "How sick is the patient?" Is this patient someone who really needs an agent that is more effective than a mesalamine agent, or perhaps combination therapy with an oral and topical mesalamine therapy?

The second question I ask is, "Where is the patient's inflammation located?" This is perhaps one of the most important issues when choosing to use mesalamine therapies in patients with inflammatory bowel disease (IBD). While all of the various therapies rely on the mesalamine component to be the anti-inflammatory, they all have different delivery mechanisms, and it is important to understand where the drug is supposed to release, and then target it appropriately to the patient (Figure 39-1).[1]

For example, patients who have small bowel CD, regardless of whether they have colonic disease as well, are best served by using Pentasa. Pentasa releases by moisture, guaranteeing release within the small intestine. Pentasa does reach the colon, and it is effective in patients with Crohn's colitis and UC as well. Personally, I find Pentasa to be the best tolerated of the mesalamine agents, and, if a patient is having difficulty tolerating some of the other agents, they will often end up on Pentasa. While it used to be a rather large number of pills (16), the 500 mg formulation has allowed us to use 6 to 8 pills to give 3 to 4 g daily. While the labeling is for 4-times-a-day dosing, I typically dose it bid (twice a day), and have not found any difference in efficacy or tolerance.

For patients who have disease located only in the colon, or perhaps at the very end of the ileum and the colon, then it is appropriate to use one of the pH-release agents such as Asacol or Lialda. Asacol currently comes as 400 mg tablets, and, while the standard

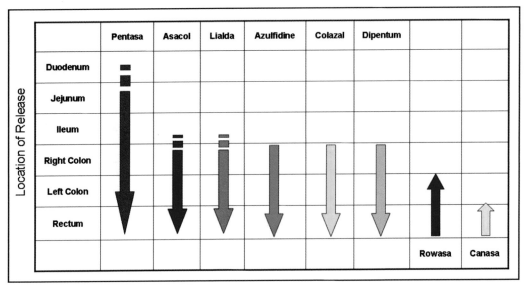

Figure 39-1. Location of medication release for mesalamine-based products.

dose is felt to be 6 pills a day, many of us use 8 to 12 pills for patients who have more aggressive disease. It is still unclear whether there is truly a dose response above 2.4 g, although sicker patients often will use higher doses of mesalamine to get better. Though the labeling is for tid (3 times a day), I usually dose Asacol bid as well to improve patient convenience and compliance.

Lialda is marketed as once-a-day dosing of 2 or 4 pills. Each pill contains 1.2 g of mesalamine. It has only been on the market for less than a year, but in my limited post-market experience with this agent, I find it to be effective at 2 to 3 pills daily. While it can be dosed bid, it is probably unnecessary to do so.[2] In the case of both Asacol and Lialda, there is the need for the bowel to reach a pH of 7 in order for the agent to release. If patients are passing tablets entirely whole or if the agent is ineffective, it is advisable to try switching to a different delivery system of mesalamine rather than just between these two agents, which have the same initial delivery. Some patients will develop diarrhea or other side effects to the coating on the Asacol or Lialda and not to some of the other delivery systems, so it is always wise to try switching between delivery systems if patients are not responding or perhaps having an adverse reaction. Obviously, a severe adverse reaction would limit the ability to use any mesalamine agents.

Colonic disease, whether the problem is ulcerative or Crohn's colitis, can be treated with any of the agents mentioned above, but the azo-bond drugs, such as Colazal (Salix Pharmaceuticals, Inc., Morrisville, NC), Dipentum (UCB, Inc., Brussels, Belgium), and Azulfidine (Pharmacia & Upjohn, Bridgewater, NJ) are specifically targeting the large intestine. Again, I dose these agents bid, although some patients prefer to use them 3 to 4 times a day due to the number of pills. In the case of Colazal, I typically give 4 pills bid and may back down to 3 pills bid when patients are in remission. Azulfidine is tricky to dose, as you have to start at a low dose (perhaps 1 g daily) and increase the dose slowly over the ensuing week or so. Dipentum also should initially be dose titrated to 1 to 2 g daily, as many patients get diarrhea with this medication. I prefer Dipentum in patients

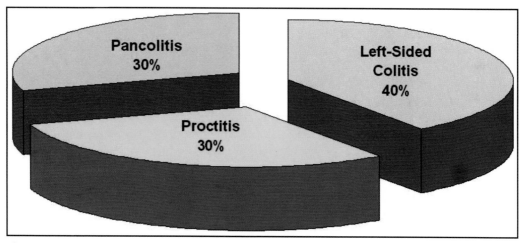

Figure 39-2. Location of disease at diagnosis in patients with ulcerative colitis.

with distal left-sided disease who have a constipation-predominant presentation. There is the thought that perhaps the diarrhea-inducing effect allows the mesalamine to reach the distal colon (or perhaps just relieves the feeling of constipation that the patient suffers from).

Topical therapies are perhaps the most overlooked agents in the approach to treating patients with UC, especially distal colitis, which can be the only location in up to 70% of patients (Figure 39-2). UC always starts in the rectum and works proximally, so one could argue that all patients should be on topical therapy. In reality, patients who just have proctitis are often most rapidly and effectively treated with mesalamine suppository (Canasa; Axcan Pharma US, Inc., Birmingham, AL).[3] Dosed at bedtime or bid, these are very effective in getting symptoms down very quickly. Patients who have proctitis but then extend proximally will often still note a benefit from including Canasa as part of their regimen, both for induction and maintenance therapy.

In patients for whom the inflammation extends beyond the rectum, mesalamine enemas (Rowasa) are also very effective.[4] These are usually dosed at bedtime, as patients may have trouble holding them during the day. Some patients find that they can use half a dose and hold the agent better. Again, these are very effective in induction and maintenance of remission. Some patients may be able to just use the enemas once or twice weekly to maintain their remission.

Luckily, the mesalamine agents are all extremely safe. Sulfasalazine has numerous safety concerns due to the sulfa moiety, and, as a result, the monitoring of blood counts, renal, and hepatic function needs to be more frequent with this agent. The non–sulfa-containing agents have very few serious adverse reactions other than idiosyncratic reactions. Patients who have a strange reaction such as a hepatitis, pericarditis, pleuritis, or pancreatitis would probably best be served without any of these agents.

There has been ongoing debate about whether there is an increased rate of interstitial nephritis in patients who are receiving mesalamine products. As the rates of interstitial nephritis are extraordinarily low, it may be difficult to know for sure whether this is truly an instigating agent in the rare cases. Nevertheless, it is wise to check renal function within 6 months of starting therapy, and then perhaps yearly afterwards. Checking urine eosinophils and sediment in patients who have suspicion of renal dysfunction can be considered.

The agent that induces remission is often the one we use to maintain remission in patients with UC and CD. Some patients prefer not to use topical therapy long term, but there is an evidence base suggesting that they are effective in the maintenance of remission, even when used intermittently throughout the week. Unfortunately, many doctors seem to shy away from even prescribing these agents, which are highly effective in patients with difficult refractory cases.

References

1. Cohen RD. Review article: evolutionary advances in the delivery of aminosalicylates for the treatment of ulcerative colitis. *Aliment Pharmacol Ther.* 2006;24(3):465-474.
2. Kamm MA, Sandborn WJ, Gassull M, et al. Once-daily, high-concentration MMX mesalamine in active ulcerative colitis. *Gastroenterology.* 2007;132(1):66-75.
3. Cohen RD, Woseth DM, Thisted RA, Hanauer SB. A meta-analysis and overview of the literature on treatment options for left-sided ulcerative colitis and ulcerative proctitis. *Am J Gastroenterol.* 2000;95(5):1263-1276.
4. Hanauer S, Good LI, Goodman MW, et al. Long-term use of mesalamine (Rowasa) suppositories in remission maintenance of ulcerative proctitis. *Am J Gastroenterol.* 2000;95(7):1749-1754.

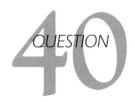

Do Probiotics Have a Role in Treating Inflammatory Bowel Disease Patients?

Joshua R. Korzenik, MD

Probiotics hold the promise of a therapy for inflammatory bowel disease (IBD), which could be effective, treat the underlying pathophysiology, and be free of adverse events. Many individuals with ulcerative colitis (UC) or Crohn's disease (CD) embrace this approach, and a substantial percentage use probiotics, often without the knowledge of their healthcare team. Unfortunately, each assertion of the hope of probiotics remains unproven, but they also have not been disproved. To date, most of the studies examining a therapeutic benefit, and there have not been many, have failed to demonstrate clinical efficacy. The field of probiotics in IBD remains in its infancy so that a clinician acts in a cloud of uncertainty in trying to determine if probiotics are beneficial, to select an appropriate probiotic or an optimal dose, and to be certain that no harm is being done.

The role of gut flora in both CD and UC has been increasingly appreciated as central to their pathophysiology. With the similarities of bacterial infections to IBD, numerous specific bacteria have been advanced as the causative agent in IBD (such as *Mycobacterium paratuberculosis* in CD), but after further scrutiny, none remain as serious candidates. Until recently, the mucosal inflammatory response was considered a nonspecific reaction to commensal gut flora. Non–culture-based techniques have begun to describe the human gut biome in greater detail and suggest more specific dysbioses or pathogenic alterations of flora, which may be related to the fundamental pathophysiology of these diseases. A specific dysbiosis describing a disease-associated bacterial fingerprint has not been consistently identified for either disease, though a variety of shifts in flora have been suggested, particularly in CD. Recent studies[1] have shown that the flora from patients with CD has a reduced diversity, generally with a decrease in the bacterial division Firmicutes, with some studies suggesting an increase in Bacteroides (though others suggest a decrease) and a decrease in *Clostridial* species. Specific bacteria have been identified as associated with CD, such as enteroadherent enteroinvasive *E. coli*. While found more frequently in patients with IBD, their role in pathogenesis remains unproven and uncertain.

Even if a clear dysbiosis is identified in either UC or CD, numerous unresolved issues persist about the potential role of probiotics to address a dysbiosis in IBD. Firstly, could the administration of live bacteria correct this altered flora to produce a clinical benefit in either disease? Secondly, even if a dysbiosis cannot be directly or completely corrected with bacterial supplementation, do probiotics still generate important physiologic effects to provide a therapeutic benefit in IBD? Several beneficial actions of probiotics have been suggested,[2] including an improvement in gut barrier function (improving intestinal integrity and decreasing permeability), augmenting immune function, displacing pathogenic bacteria (which may be important in stimulating the inflammatory response), increasing interleukin 10 (IL-10) production, and increasing T-regulatory cell activity. However, not all probiotics have similar benefits, and most have not been studied for potential clinical benefit. Of interest and potential importance, essentially none of the functions ascribed to probiotics as beneficial in IBD are similar to the actions of standard therapies utilized for the treatment of IBD, such as steroids and immunosuppressants (azathioprine, 6-mercaptopurine [6-MP], infliximab, adalimumab, certolizumab, natalizumab).

The selection of probiotics would ideally be guided by appropriate translational and clinical studies. Most probiotics purchased by patients have little or no investigations to support the claims of a health effect, and they are even less likely to have a benefit in IBD. The field is not monitored or regulated, so the manufacturing process sometimes produces bacteria different from the label with different doses and unknown effects. Furthermore, the randomized, placebo-controlled trials in this area have been largely flawed or negative. The most positive study of probiotics in IBD is a randomized controlled trial of VSL#3 performed in pouchitis, which was an important proof of principal study for the field.[3] VSL#3 is a mixture of 8 different bacteria, most of which is *Streptococcus thermophilus*, as well as lesser amounts of *Bifidobacteria* and *Lactobacillus* species. This study enrolled 40 patients with chronic pouchitis who were brought into remission with antibiotics. Individuals were then randomized to placebo or VSL#3 at a dose of 900 billion bacteria twice daily. (As a reference, most other probiotics doses range from 500,000 to 30 billion bacteria daily. One gram of stool contains between 100 billion bacteria to 1 trillion bacteria.) In this study, all 20 patients taking the placebo flared within 9 months, while only 3/20 flared while taking the VSL#3. While a dramatic result, these results may not be generalizable to UC or CD. Milder benefits have been suggested in studies of VSL#3 in CD or UC. In addition, pouchitis is the most antibiotic-sensitive subgroup of IBD, and those with a pouch also have a smaller reservoir of bacteria, possibly making pouchitis an easier therapeutic target for probiotics than CD or UC.

Another probiotic extensively studied for the use in IBD (and approved for treatment for UC in Germany) is Nissle 1917. This *Escherichia coli* (*E. coli*) strain was isolated by a German army surgeon from the stool of a soldier who remained healthy during a severe outbreak of Shigellosis that either killed or sickened numerous other soldiers in his unit. This strain has been studied for the treatment of flares of UC as well as the maintenance of remission both using mesalamine as the comparator. In the acute treatment trial (116 patients total), 44 patients (75%) receiving mesalamine achieved remission compared with 39 (68%) receiving *E. coli* Nissle 1917.[4] In a 12-month maintenance study,[5] relapses were seen in 40/110 (36.4%) patients in the *E. coli* Nissle 1917 group compared to 38/112 (33.9%) in the mesalamine group (p = 0.003). These studies have been criticized for several study design issues, including the use of a relatively low dose of mesalamine (1.2 g/day in one study and 1.5 g/day in another).

One of the most rigorously designed and conducted studies determined the strain selection after testing over 1400 strains for a variety of likely beneficial characteristics, such as the ability to survive through acid and bile, and the capacity to adhere to colonic mucosa. Two strains selected—*Bifidobacterium infantis* and *Lactobacillus salivarius*—were individually compared to placebo in a 12-month trial for the maintenance of remission after individuals were brought into remission by steroids.[6] No differences were seen between any of the 3 groups (2 probiotic groups and the placebo group) at the end of 1 year, with approximately 50% in each group flaring. This trial, which had high hopes as a clear proof of principle study in UC, failed to demonstrate any benefit. A number of other studies have failed to demonstrate a benefit of probiotics in IBD as well, including a postoperative prevention of recurrence trial[7] using *Lactobacillus johnsonii* and a pediatric maintenance of remission trial in CD using *Lactobacillus GG*.[8]

Probiotics are eagerly advocated by patients and physicians in part because, even if their benefit is unproven, the use of probiotics appears to be without any serious or even mild adverse events. While this assertion is likely to be the case, the safety is not established. Several studies in animal models of IBD have suggested a lesser benefit of *Lactobacillus* than *Bifidobacteria* species, and when used in combination, *Lactobacillus* may reduce the benefit demonstrated by *Bifidobacteria* species. More worrisome, though of uncertain significance for the IBD population, was a recent randomized trial[9] of a probiotic mixture for individuals with severe acute pancreatitis, which found a higher rate of transfer to the intensive care unit (ICU), surgical intervention, and a significantly higher death rate in the group randomized to probiotics. In this large trial, 24/152 patients (16%) in the probiotics group died, compared with 9/145 (6%) in the placebo group (relative risk [RR] 2·53, 95% CI 1·22–5·25). This study should not be interpreted to suggest that probiotics are a potentially life-threatening therapy in IBD. Furthermore, probiotics are not a monolithic therapy, but different probiotics have different physiologic effects. The long track record and extensive use of probiotics underscore a strong safety record. However, the use of certain probiotics might have unrecognized, unintended consequences in the IBD population.

So what can be concluded about the research done to date in the use of probiotics in IBD, and what can be recommended? First, some caveats should be clear: not all probiotics are similar, and they do not necessarily share physiologic effects. If a benefit may exist of a particular probiotic in IBD, dosing is critical. Both of these issues suggest that taking a random mixture or single species purchased at a health food store or elsewhere has a low likelihood of benefiting the patient. A straight evidenced-based approach to probiotics would direct a practitioner to limit the use of probiotics to certain subgroups of patients (those with pouchitis or possibly UC) and the use of a limited set of probiotics (VSL#3, which is available in the United States, or Nissle 1917, sold in Germany as Mutaflor [Ardeypharm, Germany]). Even these benefits may not be applicable to a set of patients within these subgroups that may differ from those studied. The promise of probiotics remains unproven, and their broad use cannot be advocated. A selective approach in a relatively small subset of patients would appear reasonable, as long as the individuals understand the limited nature of the data, the conceivable possibility of unintended adverse consequences, and the primitive state of the knowledge of the gut biome. Hopefully, in the near future, advances in our ability to manipulate the intestinal environment will guide the broader use of these therapies in individuals with IBD.

References

1. Frank DN, St Amand AL, Feldman RA, Boedeker EC, Harpaz N, Pace NR. Molecular-phylogentic characterization of microbial community imbalances in human inflammatory bowel diseases. *PNAS.* 2007;104(34):13780-13785.
2. Sartor RB. Therapeutic manipulation of the enteric microflora in inflammatory bowel diseases: antibiotics, probiotics, and prebiotics. *Gastroenterology.* 2004;126(6):1620-1633.
3. Gionchetti P, Rizzello F, Venturi A, et al. Oral bacteriotherapy as maintenance treatment in patients with chronic pouchitis: a double-blind, placebo-controlled trial. *Gastroenterology.* 2000;119(2):305-309.
4. Rembacken BJ, Snelling AM, Hawkey PM, Chalmers DM, Axon AT. Non-pathogenic Escherichia coli versus mesalazine for the treatment of ulcerative colitis: a randomised trial. *Lancet.* 1999;354(9179):635-639.
5. Kruis W, Schutz E, Fric P, Fixa B, Judmaiers G, Stolte M. Double blind comparison of an oral Escherichia coli preparation and mesalazine in maintaing remission of ulcerative colitis. *Aliment Pharmacol Ther.* 1997;11(5):853-853.
6. Shanahan F, Guraner F, von Wright A, Vilpponene-Salmela T, O'Donoghue D, Kiely B. A one year, randomised, double-blind, placebo controlled trial of a lactobacillus or a bidifobacterium probiotic for maintenance of steroid-induced remission of ulcerative colitis. *Gastroenterology.* 2006;130 (suppl 2):A44
7. Marteau P, Lemann M, Seksik P, et al. Ineffectiveness of Lactobacillus johnsonii LA1 for prophylaxis of post-operative recurrence in Crohn's disease: a randomised, double blind, placebo controlled GETAID trial. *Gut.* 2006;55(6):842-847.
8. Bousvaros A, Guandalini S, Baldasano S, et al. A randomized, double-blind trial of Lactobacillus GG versus placebo in addition to standard maintenance therapy for children with Crohn's disease. *Inflamm Bowel Dis.* 2005;11(9):833-839.
9. Besselink M, Santvoort Hv, Buskens E, et al. Probiotic prophylaxis in predicted severe acute pancreatitis: a randomised, double-blind, placebo-controlled trial. *Lancet.* 2008;371(9613):651-659.

41

WHAT IS YOUR FIRST LINE APPROACH TO THE DIAGNOSIS AND TREATMENT OF PATIENTS WITH PERIANAL CROHN'S DISEASE?

David A. Schwartz, MD

Perianal Crohn's disease (CD), or more specifically, fistulizing CD, is one of the more dreaded complications for patients with this disease. If not treated aggressively from the onset, it can often negatively affect the patient's quality of life in a dramatic way, secondary to pain or incontinence. In the worst cases, it can even result in proctectomy. In order to prevent these potential outcomes, I approach Crohn's patients with perianal disease using a modified "top-down" approach employing a multi-modality (radiology, surgery, and medicine) treatment strategy (Figure 41-1).

When a patient presents with a possible fistula, I start by reassessing their perianal disease. Fistulas should be divided into complex and simple fistulas in order to plan treatment. A simple fistula is a superficial, inter-sphincteric, or low trans-sphincteric fistula with only one opening. It is neither associated with an abscess nor does it connect to an adjacent structure. A complex fistula is one that involves more of the anal sphincters (ie, high trans-sphincteric, extra-sphincteric, or supra-sphincteric), has multiple openings, "horseshoes" (crossing the midline either anteriorly or posteriorly), is associated with a perianal abscess, and/or connects to an adjacent structure such as the vagina or bladder.

Delineation of the fistulizing process is done first with a thorough physical exam, but it is important to also image the patient with either magnetic resonance imaging (MRI) or endorectal ultrasound (EUS). Physical exam is not very accurate in this setting because of all of the pain, induration, and scarring associated with perianal CD. Studies have shown that either MRI or EUS are highly accurate in assessing perianal CD.[1]

Creating this virtual roadmap of the patients' perianal disease for the surgeon is important to do prior to starting treatment because several studies have demonstrated that failure to fully recognize and treat all of the perianal process (ie, abscess and fistu-

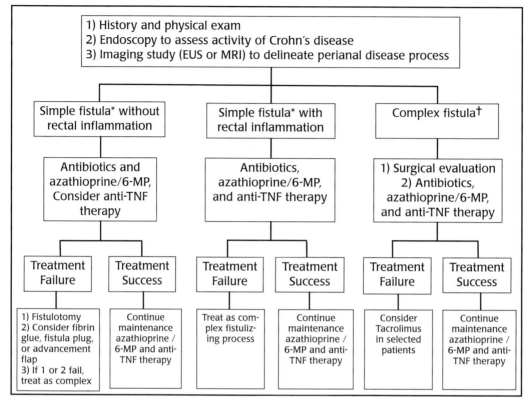

1) History and physical exam
2) Endoscopy to assess activity of Crohn's disease
3) Imaging study (EUS or MRI) to delineate perianal disease process

Simple fistula* without rectal inflammation	Simple fistula* with rectal inflammation	Complex fistula†
Antibiotics and azathioprine/6-MP, Consider anti-TNF therapy	Antibiotics, azathioprine/6-MP, and anti-TNF therapy	1) Surgical evaluation 2) Antibiotics, azathioprine/6-MP, and anti-TNF therapy

Treatment Failure	Treatment Success	Treatment Failure	Treatment Success	Treatment Failure	Treatment Success
1) Fistulotomy 2) Consider fibrin glue, fistula plug, or advancement flap 3) If 1 or 2 fail, treat as complex	Continue maintenance azathioprine / 6-MP and anti-TNF therapy	Treat as complex fistuliz-ing process	Continue maintenance azathioprine / 6-MP and anti-TNF therapy	Consider Tacrolimus in selected patients	Continue maintenance azathioprine / 6-MP and anti-TNF therapy

Figure 41-1. Treatment Algorithm. *A simple fistula is a superficial, inter-sphincteric or low trans-sphincteric fistula with only one opening, and it is neither associated with an abscess nor connects to an adjacent structure. †A complex fistula is one that involves more of the anal sphincters (ie, high trans-sphincteric, extra-sphincteric, or supra-sphincteric), has multiple openings, "horseshoes" (crossing the midline either anteriorly or posteriorly), is associated with a perianal abscess, and/or connects to an adjacent structure such as the vagina or bladder.

las branches) can result in a simple fistula becoming a complex fistula and/or recurrent fistulas or abscesses.[2] Once a fistula becomes complex, the chance for complete closure of the fistula is dramatically reduced.[2] Because of this, once a fistula becomes a complex fistula, the goal of treatment becomes primarily one of symptom control (ie, cessation of drainage), and not complete closure or fibrosis of the tract. So in essence, you may have only one shot to get a fistula to close completely. Imaging with EUS or MRI increases your odds of accomplishing this goal.

At this point, I send the patient to the surgeon for an exam under anesthesia (EUA). By using the imaging "roadmap," the surgeon can make sure all abscesses are drained and setons are placed in all of the fistulas prior to starting treatment. Retrospective studies have shown that seton placement prior to starting infliximab reduces the rate of fistula recurrence dramatically (44% versus 79%).[3] Setons work by preventing the premature closure of the cutaneous opening of the fistula tract prematurely (ie, prior to the time when fistula inactivity occurs) (Figure 41-2).

Once drainage has been established, it is time to institute medical therapy. Because of the potential negative outcomes associated with perianal CD, I start anti-tumor necrosis

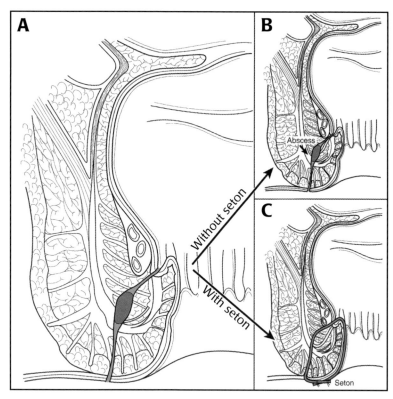

Figure 41-2. Typical trans-sphincteric fistulas prior to treatment (A). Without seton placement prior to anti-TNF therapy, one gets premature closure of cutaneous openings and abscess formation (B). Seton placement prior to initiation of medical treatment prevents abscess formation by allowing fistula to drain until inflammation is absent (C).

factor alpha (anti-TNF-α) antibodies at the onset along with immunomodulators (azathioprine or 6-mercaptopurine [6-MP]) and an antibiotic (ciprofloxacin or metronidazole) (see Figure 41-1). Similar to the rationale for the "top-down" approach (using anti-TNF-α therapy before steroids or proven failure of oral thiopurines) for luminal CD, this modified "top-down" approach aims to aggressively treat the fistulizing disease from the onset, with the maximum amount of treatment currently available in order to achieve healing and prevent the complications that can occur with perianal CD. Studies have shown that anti-TNF-α treatment with infliximab or adalimumab results in complete cessation of drainage in about 50% to 60% of patients treated, and maintenance of cessation of fistula drainage throughout a year in about 30% to 40% of the patients who respond to the initial treatment.[4-6] In ACCENT II (A Crohn's Disease Clinical Trial Evaluating Infliximab in a New Long-Term Treatment Regimen), the infliximab fistula maintenance trial, infliximab was used to maintain fistula closure over the course of a year.[5] In this trial, the 195 patients who were considered responders (≥ 50% reduction in draining fistulas) at week 14 to the initial induction sequence of infliximab 5 mg/kg at zero, 2, and 6 weeks were randomized to receive either 5 mg/kg or placebo every 8 weeks. At week 54, 36% of patients who were on maintenance infliximab had complete cessation of drainage of all of their fistulas, compared to only 19% of patients in the placebo cohort (p = 0.009).

Fistula healing was studied as a secondary endpoint in the adalimumab maintenance trial, CHARM (Crohn's Trial of the Fully Human Antibody Adalimumab for Remission Maintenance).[6] Complete fistula closure at week 56 was seen in 33% of the treated group (combined 40 mg weekly and every-other-week adalimumab dosing arms) compared with 13% in the placebo arm ($p = .016$). The response was durable. In the patients who demonstrated fistula closure at week 26, all maintained fistula closure at week 56.

Another common approach (especially those with simple fistulas) is to use antibiotics (Cipro [Bayer Healthcare, Pittsburgh, PA] or metronidazole) as a bridge to immunomodulator treatment in patients with Crohn's perianal fistulas.[7] A prospective open label trial of 52 patients with Crohn's perianal fistulas compared those patients treated only with ciprofloxacin or metronidazole for 8 weeks to those patients who transitioned or were already on azathioprine at a dose of 2 to 2.5 mg/kg/day. Although the results at week 8 were similar between the 2 groups, those that were maintained on azathioprine had a higher "response" rate by week 20 (48% versus 15%; $p = 0.03$).

Usually, fistulas will stop draining after 2 to 6 weeks of treatment if anti-TNF-α therapy is used. Currently, the typical practice is to remove the setons at this point. It is my practice, however, to use imaging with EUS to determine when to remove the setons. EUS and MRI studies have shown that the internal portion of the fistula remains active long after the fistula stops draining. Therefore, I leave the seton in until EUS demonstrates fistula inactivity. The same approach could be utilized with MRI as well. We have shown in a retrospective study[8] and in a small randomized prospective trial[9] that utilizing EUS to guide therapy in this way improves the long-term treatment success rate with a combination of medical and surgical therapy.

References

1. Schwartz DA, Wiersema MJ, Dudiak KM, et al. A comparison of endoscopic ultrasound, magnetic resonance imaging, and exam under anesthesia for evaluation of Crohn's perianal fistulas. *Gastroenterology.* 2001;121(5):1064-1072.
2. Williamson PR, Hellinger MD, Larach SW, Ferrara A. Twenty-year review of the surgical management of perianal Crohn's disease. *Diseases of the Colon & Rectum.* 1995;38(4):389-392.
3. Regueiro M, Mardini H. Treatment of perianal fistulizing Crohn's disease with infliximab alone or as an adjunct to exam under anesthesia with seton placement. *Inflamm Bowel Dis.* 2003;9(2):98-103.
4. Present DH, Rutgeerts P, Targan S, et al. Infliximab for the treatment of fistulas in patients with Crohn's disease. *N Eng J Med.* 1999;340(18):1398-1405.
5. Sands B, Van Deventer S, Bernstein C. Long-term treatment of fistulizing Crohn's disease: Response to infliximab in ACCENT II trials through 54 weeks. *Gastroenterology.* 2002;122:A81.
6. Colombel JF, Sandborn WJ, Rutgeerts P, et al. Adalimumab for maintenance of clinical response and remission in patients with Crohn's disease: the CHARM trial. *Gastroenterology.* 2007;132(1):52-65.
7. Dejaco C, Harrer M, Waldhoer T, Miehsler W, Vogelsang H, Reinisch W. Antibiotics and azathioprine for the treatment of perianal fistulas in Crohn's disease. *Aliment Pharmacol Ther.* 2003;18(11-12):1113-1120.
8. Schwartz DA, White CM, Wise PE, Herline AJ. Use of endoscopic ultrasound to guide combination medical and surgical therapy for patients with Crohn's perianal fistulas. *Inflamm Bowel Dis.* 2005;11(8):727-732.
9. Spradlin NM, Wise PE, Herline AJ, Muldoon RL, Rosen M, Schwartz DA. A randomized prospective trial of endoscopic ultrasound to guide combination medical and surgical treatment for Crohn's perianal fistulas. *Am J Gastroenterol.* 2008;103(10):2527-2535.

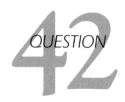

HOW DO YOU HANDLE AN INFLAMMATORY BOWEL DISEASE PATIENT WITH CLOSTRIDIUM DIFFICILE INFECTION?

David G. Binion, MD

CLOSTRIDIUM DIFFICILE INFECTION IN PATIENTS WITH IBD

At the present time, it is not uncommon to encounter inflammatory bowel disease (IBD), Crohn's disease (CD), or ulcerative colitis (UC) patients experiencing clinical flare, and in the course of evaluation, finding a positive stool ELISA (Enzyme-Linked ImmunoSorbent Assay) test for *Clostridium difficile* (*C. difficile*). In past years, *C. difficile* was felt to be a rare contributing factor for flare in the setting of IBD, but this is no longer the case. It is essential for clinicians to be aware of *C. difficile* and its potential role in the unexpected deterioration of a stable IBD patient in remission, as well as its potential contribution to a refractory flare, unresponsive to increased immunosuppression.

C. difficile is an enteric pathogen responsible for a spectrum of illnesses ranging from mild diarrhea to fulminant colitis, leading to sepsis and potentially death. *C. difficile*-associated disease has doubled in North America over the past 5 years.[1] Patients with IBD appear to be at an increased risk of acquiring *C. difficile*, as well as having increased morbidity and mortality from this pathogen.[2] Given that the symptoms of *C. difficile*-associated disease mimic those of IBD colitis flare, it is essential that clinicians aggressively identify co-infection with this pathogen in IBD patients experiencing disease flare. *C. difficile* infection must be treated with antibiotics targeting the bacteria, and the use of nonspecific immunosuppressive agents for colitis flare in the setting of a bacterial infection of the colon may worsen the disease process.

THE SPECTRUM OF CLOSTRIDIUM DIFFICILE IN IBD

The rise in *C. difficile* infections, and their increasing impact on patients with IBD, became apparent in the years after 2000. Data from our center has demonstrated a significant rise in the number of IBD patients infected between 2001 and 2005.[3] Most importantly, there was a disproportionate rise in the percentage of IBD patients within the total number of *C. difficile* infections occurring at our institution. The percentage of IBD patients within the total number of *C. difficile* infections rose from 4% in 2004 to 16% in 2005. Rodeman et al from Washington University also found that IBD patients represented a disproportionate number of the individuals contracting *C. difficile*.[4] These experiences from individual centers were also confirmed using the National Inpatient Sample, which showed that IBD patients had significantly more morbidity and mortality as a result of *C. difficile* infection.[2] *C. difficile* infections occurred in 4.6% of the IBD patients followed at our institution in 2005, and 10% of the IBD patients at our institution have had a documented episode of *C. difficile* infection during their lifetime.[3]

IMPACT OF *CLOSTRIDIUM DIFFICILE* ON IBD

Among the IBD patients with a documented *C. difficile* infection during the years 2004 and 2005, 60% required hospitalization, and 20% underwent colectomy due to refractory colitis.[3] The infection appears to be synergistic with IBD flare, and both the infection and the resultant flare will require treatment.

DIAGNOSIS OF *CLOSTRIDIUM DIFFICILE* IN PATIENTS WITH IBD

Diagnosis of *C. difficile* infection is routinely carried out with stool ELISAs for the presence of bacterial toxins A and/or B. Although these assays are extremely specific for the presence of the infection, they have limited sensitivity. In our experience during the year 2005, the first stool ELISA sample was able to detect 54% of the patients with documented infection.[3] Four stool samples raised the detection rate to approximately 90%. Therefore, it is essential to process multiple specimens in order to accurately detect infection.

Among the IBD patients who contracted *C. difficile* in 2005, we found that 61% had had a documented exposure to antibiotics within the preceding 2 months, with the quinolone ciprofloxacin being the most commonly associated antibiotic.[3] Therefore, 39% of IBD patients with proven *C. difficile* developed the infection with no known exposure to recent broad spectrum antibiotics, which again challenges past dogma regarding traditional risk factors for the contraction of this infection. Likewise, the vast majority of IBD patients (78%) were non-institutionalized outpatients at the time of *C. difficile* infection, again suggesting that a prior history of IBD is in itself a risk factor for the development of *C. difficile*-associated disease.

Among the IBD patients who ultimately developed *C. difficile* infection, 91% had a history of IBD colitis (either UC or Crohn's involvement of the colon).[3] Multivariate logistic regression analysis demonstrated that a prior history of colitis was significantly associated with the development of *C. difficile* infection. The use of maintenance immunosuppression, but not 5-aminosalicylic acid (5-ASA) use or infliximab maintenance, was also associated with infection with *C. difficile*.

The classic endoscopic appearance of *C. difficile* is a pseudomembranous colitis, which may be identified in up to 50% of otherwise healthy individuals who contract this infection. In the IBD patient population, pseudomembranous colitis is rarely seen, thus making identification of the infection even more difficult.[3] In our cohort of IBD patients who were diagnosed with *C. difficile* in 2005, pseudomembranes were not identified in any of the patients who underwent endoscopy or who required surgical intervention. In addition, the classic histologic features of a fibrinopurulent eruption were also not seen on histology. Thus, stool evaluation for the presence of toxin is essential to make the diagnosis.

TREATMENT OF *CLOSTRIDIUM DIFFICILE* IN IBD PATIENTS

The key principles for successfully treating *C. difficile* infection involve limiting the use of broad spectrum antibiotics, which will alter intestinal flora and favor the growth of the pathogen. The treatment of *C. difficile* has emphasized the use of metronidazole, and studies from 10 years prior demonstrated a success rate of 90% with this antibiotic. More recent data has suggested that 50% of cases will fail to respond clinically with this agent.[5] In our institutional experience, the hospitalization rates for *C. difficile* infection remained stable during the years 2004, 2005, and 2006, while the rate of colectomy fell. This corresponded to a switch to the use of oral vancomycin as the major treatment strategy for *C. difficile*.[6]

Finally, *C. difficile* infection will frequently result in a concomitant exacerbation of the underlying IBD colitis. This will require the use of immunosuppressive agents for the simultaneous colitis flare. The modification of intravenous (IV) corticosteroid dosage may be considered in this setting, as these agents are particularly effective in blunting humoral immune responses, while the successful clearance of a *C. difficile* infection requires mounting an antibody response against *C. difficile* toxin A. Therefore, using 50 mg of IV hydrocortisone every 8 hours (as opposed to 100 mg every 8 hours) has become our favored approach for treating IBD flare in the setting of hospitalized patients with *C. difficile*.[6] The reduction in the colectomy rates for the *C. difficile*-infected patients at our institution between the years 2004 and 2006 was paralleled by a deliberate attempt to limit and reduce the dosages of IV steroids in all patients with either documented or suspected *C. difficile* who required hospitalization for the treatment of their colitis. In individuals who are failing to resolve despite appropriate antibiotics against *C. difficile* and corticosteroids, anti-tumor necrosis factor alpha (TNF-α) antibody therapy with infliximab has been successfully used in this population as well. Finally, the use of probiotic agents including *Saccharomyces boulardii* and *lactobacillus* strains can be considered, but there is a lack of specific data regarding the efficacy of these agents in the IBD population that has been infected by *C. difficile*.

In addition, having IBD patients maintain oral intake (if possible) will be an important adjunct, as the intestinal flora will be dependent on non-digestible starches coming through the gastrointestinal (GI) tract to maintain their viability. Furthermore, withholding oral intake may actually provide a growth advantage for anaerobic flora, including *C. difficile*.

SPECIAL CLINICAL ISSUE REGARDING *CLOSTRIDIUM DIFFICILE* IN IBD

IBD patients may be challenged by unique clinical scenarios involving *C. difficile* infection. These may include small bowel infection, the so-called *C. difficile* enteritis.[7] We have encountered this as an early complication in patients who have undergone colectomy either for the initial treatment of fulminant IBD colitis, or as a component of staged procedures during ileoanal J pouch reconstruction. Patients may present with fever, abdominal pain, ileus, and decreased ostomy output. Computerized tomography will reveal dilated loops of edematous small intestine, and testing the ileostomy output is essential to make the diagnosis. Other unique clinical scenarios where *C. difficile* may emerge include an infection of diverted segments of the large bowel, including the rectal remnant or Hartman's pouch, or in surgically diverted colonic segments downstream from a double barrel loop ileostomy. In these settings, it is essential to use vancomycin enemas to effectively deliver antibiotic therapy to the downstream bowel that is out of continuity from orally delivered medications.

SUMMARY

IBD patients are at an increased risk of acquiring *C. difficile* infection, and they are at an increased risk of colectomy and mortality from this infection. The subgroup of IBD patients who may be at the highest risk are individuals with underlying colitis—either Crohn's colitis or UC. A high index of suspicion for this infection in IBD patients experiencing disease flare is essential, as a majority of patients will acquire the infection as outpatients, and approximately 40% may not have had exposure to broad spectrum antibiotics in the months preceding the episode. Multiple stool samples for toxin analysis are essential to confirm diagnosis in the majority of IBD patients. Treatment may start with metronidazole, but a lack of clinical response within 48 hours or a severe presentation requiring hospitalization should prompt consideration for the use of oral vancomycin as the primary treatment of *C. difficile*. Finally, a concomitant flare of the underlying IBD will frequently accompany the infection, and this will necessitate the use of immunosuppressive agents, including corticosteroids and infliximab, in addition to antibiotics in hospitalized patients with severe disease.

References

1. McDonald LC, Owings M, Jernigan D. Clostridium difficile infection in patients discharged from US short-stay hospitals, 1996-2003. *Emerg Infect Dis.* 2006;12(3):409-415.
2. Ananthakrishnan AN, McGinley EL, Binion DG. Excess hospitalization burden associated with Clostridium difficile in patients with inflammatory bowel disease. *Gut.* 2008;57(2):205-210. Epub 2007.
3. Issa M, Vijayapal A, Bajaj JS, et al. Impact of Clostridium difficile on inflammatory bowel disease. *Clin Gastroenterol Hepatol.* 2007;5(3):345-351.
4. Rodemann JF, Dubberke ER, Reske KA, Sheo DH, Stone CD. Incidence of Clostridium difficile infection in inflammatory bowel disease. *Clin Gastroenterol Hepatol.* 2007;5(3):339-344.
5. Musher DM, Aslam S, Logan N, et al. Relatively poor outcome after treatment of Clostridium difficile colitis with metronidazole. *Clin Infect Dis.* 2005;40(11):1586-1590. Epub 2005.
6. Issa M, Weber R, Otterson MF, et al. Decreasing rates of colectomy despite high rates of hospitalization in Clostridium difficile infected IBD patients: a tertiary referral center ecperience. *Gastroenterology.* 2007;132: A663.
7. Lundeen SJ, Otterson MF, Binion DG, Carman ET, Peppard WJ. Clostridium difficile enteritis: an early postoperative complication in inflammatory bowel disease patients after colectomy. *J Gastrointest Surg.* 2007;11(2):138-142.

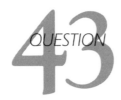

43

HOW DO YOU MANAGE MODERATE TO SEVERE DUODENAL CROHN'S DISEASE?

Charles N. Bernstein, MD and Linda Tang, MD

Previous epidemiological studies have shown that Crohn's disease (CD) is limited to the small bowel in 31% of patients. Most of the small bowel disease is located in the ileum. Isolated colonic disease (11%) and ileocecal involvement (58%) comprise the remainder of the other cases. Gastroduodenal involvement is rare, occurring in only 0.5% to 4% of all cases.[1-3] The prevalence of gastroduodenal CD is now probably higher than this as the disease entity has become more recognized over the last 20 years, particularly with patients' increased willingness to pursue upper endoscopy. There is a 20% higher incidence in males.[4] Because of proximity, CD lesions can locally erode into the pancreas or obstruct the pancreatic duct leading to pancreatitis. Hence, gastroduodenal CD should be considered if CD patients have pancreatitis.

The treatment for moderate to severe duodenal CD can be medical, endoscopic, or surgical. Similar to other treatments for CD, the objective is to avoid surgical treatment as long as possible in order to prevent short bowel syndrome and other complications related to surgical resection. The proximal duodenum, in particular, is a difficult area to resect. There is no strong evidence for proton pump inhibitors (PPI), but generally, we believe that this class of medication may be helpful in facilitating healing by reducing gastric acidity, which may be directly injurious or, at a miminum, interfere with healing. Some of the other medical therapies that can be used in duodenal CD include corticosteroids, immunomodulators like azathioprine and methotrexate (MTX), and anti-tumor necrosis factor (TNF) therapy like infliximab and adalimumab. Five-aminosalicyclic acid (5-ASA) products do not have a role in treating gastroduodenal CD. When patients have a short segment of duodenal stricture, endoscopic balloon dilatation can be very effective. When corticosteroids or balloon dilation are required, immunomodulators should be used to facilitate maintenance of remission. An alternate approach is using anti-TNF agents to settle active disease and to maintain remission, either with or without concurrent immunomodulators. In addition, surgical treatments such as stricturoplasty can be considered in cases with longer segments of duodenal strictures as an alternative to duodenal resection. Although total parenteral nutrition (TPN) and bowel rest have been used, there are no trials that support its benefit in severe CD.

Patients with obstruction secondary to duodenal CD may benefit from TPN if they have lost over 10% of their body weight and are awaiting surgery. Enteral nutrition via tube feeding, or if a patient can tolerate sufficient orally ingested quantities, is an alternate approach to supplement nutrition or to facilitate symptom reduction. Patients should use multivitamin supplementation, and calcium and vitamin D supplementation should be considered unless patients have sufficient dietary intake of these two nutrients. As the proximal duodenum is the site of iron absorption, iron deficiency should also be considered. Serum ferritin, vitamin B12, and vitamin D levels should be checked in all CD patients and replaced as necessary. For patients who live in more northern climates with reduced sun exposure, vitamin D supplementation can be considered routinely.

PROTON PUMP INHIBITORS

Generally, evidence for PPI use is lacking in the literature. Theoretically, PPIs help reduce acid and, in combination with other treatments for duodenal CD, may help with healing. PPIs are also useful because it is not always clear whether the ulcers found are secondary to CD, and a trial of PPI typically has few side effects. In one series of 17 patients with duodenal CD, 5 out of 10 patients receiving cimetidine or antacids in conjunction with prednisone had response rates lasting 2 to 9 months.[4] One interesting study suggested that acid production may be related to the length of the bowel. Shorter bowel lengths were associated with a higher degree of acid production. Thus, duodenal CD patients who undergo surgical resection of their small bowel may benefit from prophylactic PPIs.[5] While well tolerated, emerging evidence about the association of osteoporosis and hip fracture as well as *Clostridium difficile* (*C. difficile*) infections in PPI users should encourage well-done clinical trials of PPI use in gastroduodenal CD, since long-term use may not be as innocuous as we have previously considered.

AZATHIOPRINE/6-MERCAPTOPURINE

Azathioprine or its metabolite, 6-mercaptopurine (6-MP), can be used as a corticosteroid-sparing medication and as an agent to reduce anti-infliximab antibodies and potentially enhance success with anti-TNF agents. Biochemical studies suggest that azathioprine can decrease intestinal permeability, Crohn's Disease Activity Index (CDAI), and C-reactive protein (CRP) levels (all markers of active disease) in patients with CD of the upper gastrointestinal (GI) tract.[6]

CORTICOSTEROIDS

Corticosteroids can be useful in the treatment of small bowel CD, but unfortunately, like in other areas of IBD, treatment is only a short-term solution because it is associated with many side effects. It can be a useful bridge to immunomodulator therapy such as azathioprine and MTX. There have been no data assessing the effectiveness of budesonide in gastroduodenal CD. Although, based on the release profile for budesonide, it is doubtful to have a benefit.

INFLIXIMAB

Since its introduction in 1997, infliximab has revolutionalized complicated small bowel CD treatment. To date, there are 2 reports of severe duodenal CD patients who have failed previous treatment with other medical therapies and surgeries who responded to infliximab.[7,8] It is likely that adalimumab will have similar benefits to infliximab in proximal CD.

ENDOSCOPIC BALLOON DILATATION

Endoscopic balloon dilation is a viable alternative to surgery in cases where there is a short stricture length of less than 2 cm. As the length of stricture increases, so does the risk of perforation. When strictures are identified, it implies that the disease is assuming a more aggressive phenotype, and more advanced therapy such as immunomodulatory agents should be considered, even if stricture dilation is proving successful.

SURGERY

A study in 1989 by the Lahey Clinic suggested that 38.5% of patients with duodenal CD fail medical therapy and ultimately require surgery.[9] Bypass procedures such as gastrojejunostomy were previously the most common surgery for duodenal CD. Other surgeries include Roux-en-Y duodenojejunostomy. The main indication for this surgery is gastroduodenal obstruction. Unfortunately, a high percentage of CD patients with surgery have sequelae requiring further surgery. In one study of 10 patients with duodenal disease treated with surgery, 7 required 10 surgeries for marginal ulceration, obstruction at or in 1 limb of the gastrojejunostomy secondary to recurring jejunal CD, or duodenal fistula. The follow-up was 13.9 years on average.[10] Recently, stricturoplasty has fallen into favor, mainly for bowel conservation purposes. Also, the recent advances in immunosuppressive therapy have made surgery a much less sought-after solution.

Moderate to severe CD is becoming a disease that is much more recognized than in the past. Our armentarium of treatments have increased significantly, and we are significantly improving our ability to manage this disorder without resorting to surgical resection.

References

1. Nugent FW, Richmond M, Park SK. Crohn's disease of the duodenum. *Gut*. 1977;18(2):115-120.
2. Fielding JF, Toye DK, Beton DC, Cooke WT. Crohn's disease of the stomach and duodenum. *Gut*. 1970;11(12):1001-1006.
3. Reynolds HL, Stellato TA. Crohn's disease of the foregut. *Surg Clin North Am*. 2001;81(1):117-135.
4. Murray JJ, Schoetz DJ, Nugent FW, Coller JA, Veindenheimer MC. Surgical management of Crohn's disease involving the duodenum. *Am J Surg*. 1984;147(1):58-65.
5. Fielding J, Cooke WT, Williams JA. Gastric-acid secretion and duodenal ulcer in Crohn's disease. *Brit J Surg*. 1970;57(11):854.
6. Miehsler W, Püspök A, Oberhuber T, Vogelsang H. Impact of different therapeutic regimens on the outcome of patients with Crohn's disease of the upper gastrointestinal tract. *Inflamm Bowel Dis*. 2001;7(2):99-105.
7. Odashima M, Otaka M, Jin M, et al. Successful treatment of refractory duodenal Crohn's disease with infliximab. *Dig Dis Sci*. 2007;52(1):31-32.
8. Knapp A. Successful infliximab therapy for a duodenal stricture caused by Crohn's disease. *Inflamm Bowel Dis*. 2005;11(12):1123-1125.
9. Nugent FW, Roy MA. Duodenal Crohn's disease: an analysis of 89 cases. *Am J Gastroenterol*. 1989;84(3):249-254.
10. Ross TM, Fazio VW, Farmer RG. Long-term results of surgical treatment for Crohn's disease of the duodenum. *Ann Surg*. 1983;197(4):399-406.

44

WHAT IS THE NECESSARY TESTING THAT SHOULD BE PERFORMED BEFORE INITIATING BIOLOGIC THERAPY?

David T. Rubin, MD, FACG, AGAF

The current biologic therapies for inflammatory bowel disease (IBD) include 3 anti-tumor necrosis factor alpha (TNF-α) therapies (infliximab, adalimumab, certolizumab pegol), an α-4 integrin adhesion molecule inhibitor (natalizumab) for Crohn's disease (CD), and infliximab for ulcerative colitis (UC). Although these therapies have demonstrated efficacy for induction and maintenance of response and remission in patients with IBD, they are also associated with known risks, including infections. One of the most serious infections is the activation of latent mycobacterium tuberculosis (TB). From 1998 through 2001, at least 70 cases of a reactivation of latent TB in patients treated with infliximab had been reported to the Food and Drug Administration (FDA) Adverse Events Reporting System, 64 of whom had lived in areas with a higher endemic TB incidence than the United States.[1] This rate of activated TB has more recently been estimated in infliximab-treated patients in post-marketing surveillance to be 0.42/1,000.[2] The Periodic Safety Update Report of the FDA has collected 157 cases of TB in approximately 350,000 infliximab-treated IBD patients. The median duration of therapy before presentation with TB was 150 days.[3] The use of adalimumab and certolizumab pegol has also been associated with the activation of latent TB.[4] In their United States labeling of indications and safety, these drugs include the recommendation to screen for TB prior to administering therapy, and they have been updated more recently to include annual retesting while still on therapy.[5-7]

Screening for TB has traditionally been performed first by careful history and physical exam (looking for evidence of previous infection and/or exposure to an infected individual, or residing in a higher risk region of the world) and then by tuberculin skin test, in which a purified protein derivative (PPD) is administered interdermally in the forearm and inspected for the presence of a wheal 48 to 72 hours later. Patients with induration of greater than 15 mm ("low risk"), 10 mm ("moderate risk"—patients that are immigrants from high-risk countries, injection drug users, or residents or employees of prisons, jails, or nursing homes), and 5 mm ("high risk"—patients that have/had HIV, recent TB contact, a chest X-ray [CXR] consistent with prior TB, or organ transplants, and other immunocompromised patients, especially those receiving corticosteroids or other immunosuppressives) are suspected to have latent TB.[8] Positive PPD prompts CXR evaluation. If there is no evidence of active TB on CXR, latent TB is suspected, and these patients should be treated with isoniazid (INH) for 9 months prior to initiating anti-TNF therapy (but most patients can not wait that long and need to start therapy after 1 to 3 months of INH).

There are several problems with this mode of testing, including the fact that many patients with IBD are anergic, leading to falsely negative test results. Furthermore, patients previously vaccinated with Bacille Calmette Guerin (BCG) will have falsely positive PPD results. Therefore, it has been described to perform PPD with a CXR or to consider performing 2 sequential PPDs separated by one week, with the first acting as a booster for the immune reaction. Most recently, studies have shown that a blood test, the interferon-gammarelease assay (IGRA), can reliably detect latent TB without the problem of anergy or false positives with prior BCG inoculation.[9,10]

Another infection of concern is chronic hepatitis B. Limited data have demonstrated that patients with chronic hepatitis B may worsen the hepatitis infection with possible liver injury or decompensation.[11] Therefore, chronic hepatitis B is a relative contraindication for treatment with anti-TNF-α therapy. Although specific screening recommendations for IBD patients do not exist, identifying patients at risk for this infection and treatment prior to initiating therapy with anti-TNF-α therapy seems prudent.

Currently, I employ a PPD and CXR in all patients at the time of starting anti-TNF therapy, and reassess annually while patients are receiving their therapy. I use a PPD positivity threshold of 5 mm in my IBD patients. The IGRA is not yet available at our institution, but I have arranged for several patients to have this test if there are uncertain findings on their CXR and they have a negative or uninterpretable PPD result. It is expected that the IGRA technology may become more widely used in the near future, with additional validation studies in the IBD population. I assess the risk of chronic hepatitis infection in my patients, and obtain standard liver function tests and a hepatitis B surface antigen prior to treatment.

Despite the described risks of infection with natalizumab, including progressive multifocal leukoencephalopathy (PML), there are no specific screening guidelines prior to initiating therapy with this biologic therapy in CD. As with other biologic therapies, patients receiving natalizumab are monitored for the development of infection while being treated. The FDA has mandated a safety monitoring program, the TOUCH (Tysabri Outreach: Unified Commitment to Health) program.[12]

In the near future, there likely will be vaccination guidelines for patients with IBD prior to initiation with immune-suppressive therapies.

References

1. Keane J, Gershon S, Wise RP, et al. Tuberculosis associated with infliximab, a tumor necrosis factor alpha-neutralizing agent. *N Eng J Med*. 2001;345(15):1098-1104.
2. Remicade (infliximab). Data on file. Malvern, PA: Centocor, Inc; 2004.
3. Periodic Safety Update Report (PSUR): Infliximab. April 2007.

4. Colombel JF, Sandborn WJ, Rutgeerts P, et al. Adalimumab for maintenance of clinical response and remission in patients with Crohn's disease: the CHARM trial. *Gastroenterology.* 2007;132(1):52-65.
5. Remicade (infliximab) [package insert]. Malvern, PA: Centocor, Inc; 2006.
6. Humira (adalimumab) [package insert]. North Chicago, IL: Abbott Laboratories; 2008.
7. Cimzia (certolizumab pegol) [package insert]. Smyrna, GA: UCB, Inc; 2008.
8. American Thoracic Society, Centers for Disease Control and Prevention, Infectious Diseases Society of America. Controlling tuberculosis in the United States. *Am J Respir Crit Care Med.* 2005;172(9):1169-1227.
9. Mori T, Sakatani M, Yamagishi F, et al. Specific detection of tuberculosis infection: an interferon-gamma-based assay using new antigens. *Am J Resp and Crit Care.* 2004;170(1):59-64.
10. Mazurek GH, Villarino ME, CDC. Guidelines for using the QuantiFERON-TB test for diagnosing latent Mycobacterium tuberculosis infection. Centers for Disease Control and Prevention. *MMWR Recomm Rep.* 2003;52(RR-2):15-18.
11. Carroll MB, Bond MI. Use of tumor necrosis factor-alpha inhibitors with chronic hepatitis B infection. *Semin Arthritis Rheum.* 2008;3(3)8:208-217.
12. Tysabri (natalizumab) [package insert]. Cambridge, MA: Biogen Idec, Inc; 2006.

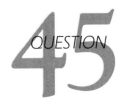

HOW DO YOU MANAGE PYODERMA GANGRENOSUM IN THE SETTING OF INFLAMMATORY BOWEL DISEASE?

Laura S. Winterfield, MD and Abrar Qureshi, MD, MPH

We follow a basic algorithm in diagnosing and treating pyoderma gangrenosum (PG) in patients with inflammatory bowel disease (IBD) (Figure 45-1).

PG is a diagnosis of exclusion, and infection must be ruled out as a first step. It is also important to consider a vasculitis, vasculopathy, or malignancy. Patients with IBD are often taking immunosuppressive medications, putting them at an increased risk of bacterial, atypical mycobacterial, and fungal infections. This makes it especially important to rule out infection in these patients.

The classic appearance of PG is an inflammatory ulcer with rolled, undermined, violaceous borders and a necrotic ulcer base (Figure 45-2). Early PG can present as small pustules or nodules that are typically very painful and may evolve rapidly into ulcers. PG can be made worse with trauma, a phenomenon known as pathergy. Because of the known association with IBD, PG should be considered in the differential diagnosis for any IBD patient who presents with tender pustules, indurated violaceous nodules, or ulcers. The possibility of pathergy should not deter you from taking a skin biopsy for histopathology and culture. PG work-up includes taking 2 skin biopsies:

1. A skin biopsy from the leading edge of the ulcer in question or from a pustule or nodule. This is then sent for bacterial, mycobacterial, and fungal stains and cultures. Note that swab cultures from open ulcers are of marginal value as they often grow colonizing bacteria that may or may not be pathogenic.

2. A second skin biopsy (also from the leading edge of the ulcer) should be sent for histopathology, including special stains (gram stain, Fite stain for acid-fast bacilli, and fungal stains).

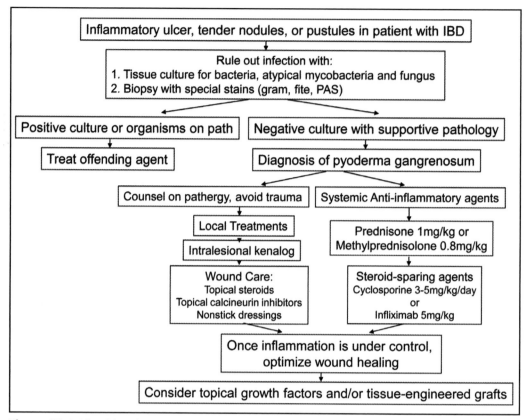

Figure 45-1. Algorithm for the diagnosis and treatment of pyoderma gangrenosum.

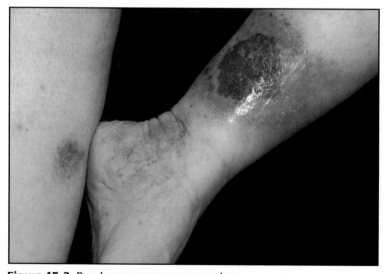

Figure 45-2. Pyoderma gangrenosum ulcer.

Once the diagnosis has been confirmed, treatment should be initiated, following a multimodal approach to decrease the inflammation, control the pain, and optimize wound healing. The first priority is to halt the progression of the disease. PG is a chronic condition and often requires long courses of immunosuppressive therapy to achieve and maintain remission:

- Corticosteroids: Almost all cases will require systemic anti-inflammatory medications, with corticosteroids as first-line therapy. The recommended starting dose is prednisone 1 mg/kg or prednisolone 0.8 mg/kg. Methyl prednisolone is a consideration in patients where prednisone absorption is not occurring optimally. A tipoff can be the lack of almost immediate pain relief upon starting prednisone, or if signs of steroid administration (eg, Cushingoid features) do not become apparent. At the same time, prophylaxis for bone and gastroinstestinal (GI) side effects should be instituted, and the addition of a steroid-sparing agent should be considered.

- Oral cyclosporine is the drug most often reported in the literature. We recommend a starting dose of 3 to 5 mg/kg, with gradual tapering of the corticosteroid dose first, once the ulcer is stable. Many of the drugs used to control IBD may also be effective for PG. In rare instances where a rapid resolution of PG is needed due to pain and discomfort, continuous infusion of intravenous (IV) cyclosporine 3 mg/kg/day can be used for 5 to 7 days. However, with access to anti-tumor necrosis factor (TNF) drugs such as infliximab, this option is not often used.

- Infliximab is the only drug that has been studied in a randomized, double-blind, placebo-controlled trial, in which it was effective in 69% of 29 patients who received it for a short term (up to 3 infusions).[1] In that small study, there was no statistically significant difference in the response rate of patients with or without coexistent IBD.

- Other drugs that have been reported to be useful in the treatment of PG include azathioprine, tacrolimus, mycophenolate mofetil, methotrexate (MTX), cyclophosphamide, thalidomide, minocycline, and dapsone.[2] With any of these drugs, appropriate monitoring for potential toxicities is imperative. We recommend frequent visits when a new therapy is introduced to evaluate for response and monitor for adverse effects.

Pain is a characteristic symptom of PG ulcers, and adequate pain control is essential to give patients the highest quality of life possible. You may work in collaboration with a pain management specialist when one is available.

Once the wound has been stabilized with adequate immunosuppressive therapy, additional agents may be added to optimize wound healing and re-epithelialization. Local wound care can further augment improvement in PG patients. This includes the local delivery of anti-inflammatory agents, and the management of the wound exudate and bacterial bioburden. In rare cases (usually very small lesions), local treatments may be sufficient to control the disease. Non-adherent dressings are preferable. Anything that sticks to the wound (eg, "wet-to-dry" dressings) may cause trauma upon removal, potentially triggering a pathergy response and causing excruciating pain for patients. Likewise, chemical debriding agents may be too irritating and induce a pathergy response. In highly exudative wounds, absorbent dressings should be used to minimize maceration of the surrounding tissue. Wound care should also include a component of antimicrobial therapy, such as topical silver or iodine-containing dressings, of which there are many available including:

- Topical steroids and/or topical tacrolimus ointment should be applied to the inflammatory wound edges with each dressing change.
- Cyclosporine drops may also be applied directly to the ulcer bed.
- Corticosteroids may be injected intralesionally into the wound edges or into new pustules or nodules as they arise. (Pathergy may be a limiting factor for this treatment.)
- Topical recombinant human platelet-derived growth factor gel may be useful when applied to a non-inflamed, clean wound bed.
- Tissue-engineered allografts may be applied to expedite wound closure and re-epithelialization. This avoids the need to create a new wound when harvesting an autologous skin graft. We also prefer to use a cyanoacrylate cement to fix the graft to surrounding skin to avoid the trauma of placing sutures.

You should also try to minimize any contributing factors that may slow down wound healing. Most PG ulcers occur on the lower extremity, where venous insufficiency and edema may contribute to poor healing. Compression wraps and/or leg elevation can help minimize the role of venous disease. You should also manage co-morbid diabetes aggressively and ensure adequate nutrition for optimal wound healing.

In the special case of peristomal PG, the literature suggests that the treatment of the underlying IBD is the most effective approach for healing the ulcers. Additionally, topical and intralesional steroids may be helpful in reducing local inflammation and expediting resolution.[3]

Surgical interventions for PG should only be considered in the context of adequate systemic anti-inflammatory therapy. In fact, elective surgical procedures for other indications should be discouraged to avoid an induction of new lesions. Removal of necrotic tissue may be warranted in some cases to reduce the risk of bacterial infection, but in most patients, this is not necessary.

References

1. Brooklyn TN, Dunnill MGS, Shetty A, et al. Infliximab for the treatment of pyoderma gangrenosum: a randomized, double blind, placebo controlled trial. *Gut.* 2006;55(4):505-509.
2. Reichrath J, Bens G, Bonowitz A, Tilgen W. Treatment recommendations for pyoderma gangrenosum: an evidence-based review of the literature based on more than 350 patients. *J Am Acad Dermatol.* 2005;53(2):273-283.
3. Yeo H, Abir F, Longo WE. Management of parastoma ulcers. *World J Gastroenterol.* 2006;12(20):3133-3137.

46

MY 25-YEAR-OLD PATIENT HAS DIFFUSE ARTHRALGIAS. CAN HE TAKE NON-STEROIDAL ANTI-INFLAMMATORY DRUGS?

Sarah N. Flier, MD and Adam S. Cheifetz, MD

The use of non-steroidal anti-inflammatory drugs (NSAIDs) in patients with inflammatory bowel disease (IBD) is the subject of some debate. In order to understand the controversy, it is important to have a basic understanding of the physiology of inflammation and the pharmacology of this class of drugs.

Tissue injury results in the release of a number of chemical factors. One such factor is arachadonic acid, a breakdown product of membrane phospholipids. The enzyme cyclooxygenase (COX) converts arachadonic acid to 3 central mediators of inflammation: prostaglandins, prostacycline, and thromboxane. The anti-inflammatory action of NSAIDs stems from their ability to inhibit the action of COX. There are 2 forms of COX, which differ primarily in their expression profiles. While cyclooxygenase 1 (COX-1) is constitutively expressed in almost all tissues and plays a role in cellular homeostasis, cyclooxygenase 2 (COX-2) is generally inducible by certain inflammatory cytokines.

The first NSAIDs available were nonselective inhibitors of both COX-1 and COX-2. Because COX-1 produces prostaglandins that protect healthy gastrointestinal (GI) mucosa, inhibiting this enzyme leads to a myriad of side effects, including but not limited to dyspepsia, gastritis, GI ulceration, enteritis, and even de novo colitis. The selective COX-2 inhibitors (coxibs) were developed to reduce inflammation without causing these toxicities.

Arthritis is the most common extraintestinal manifestation of IBD, occurring in approximately 25% of patients. However, patients with IBD also suffer the same aches and pains of daily life that affect the general population. NSAIDs are widely prescribed by general practitioners for their analgesic, anti-inflammatory, and antipyretic properties. Among rheumatologists, they are the key element in the treatment of inflammatory joint symptoms. It should come as no surprise then that many patients with IBD have taken or are considering the use of an NSAID. In one study, 42% of patients with IBD admitted to taking NSAIDs on at least one office visit over a 5-year period.[1]

In general, the effect of NSAIDs on IBD has not been carefully studied. A number of papers have reported an association between the use of NSAIDs and either the development of IBD or an exacerbation of established IBD. Still, others have found no such association. In addition to being inconclusive, many of the studies to date are limited by small sample size, retrospective design, and a lack of control for both maintenance therapy and smoking status. Furthermore, the mechanism by which NSAID use might cause or exacerbate IBD is unclear and perhaps counterintuitive. COX-2 expression has been shown to be increased in the inflamed intestinal tissue of patients with ulcerative colitis (UC) and Crohn's disease (CD), and COX-2 inhibition has been shown to effectively reduce the severity of experimental colitis. For this reason, many clinicians and investigators initially thought that NSAIDs would be beneficial in patients with IBD. On the other hand, COX-2 promotes wound healing, and one could postulate that any drug that enhances mucosal permeability would increase the exposure of the immune system to the GI flora, which is a proposed mechanism for the development of IBD.

Although earlier studies with the limitations noted above reached varying conclusions with respect to the safety of NSAIDs in IBD, more recent studies of nonselective coxibs suggest that they should be avoided when possible. In one such study of conventional NSAID use in IBD patients in clinical remission, Takeuchi et al found that 17% to 28% of the patients taking an NSAID had a clinical relapse within 2 to 9 days of initiating the drug.[2] One-third of the patients who relapsed required treatment with corticosteroids to re-induce remission. There was no difference in relapse rates between patients with UC and CD, and relapse was unlikely if the medication was tolerated for a week. Based on the second arm of their study in which patients received medications with varying types of COX inhibition, this group concluded that inhibition of both isoenzymes of COX is necessary to induce a flare. Aspirin (COX-1 inhibitor) and nimesulide (COX-2 inhibitor) appeared as safe as acetaminophen, whereas nabumetone and naproxen (nonselective COX inhibition) lead to relapse in 20% of patients.

Studies of selective COX-2 inhibitors remain controversial. Matuk et al retrospectively studied 33 patients with IBD in remission who were prescribed a selective COX-2 inhibitor.[3] Thirty-nine percent of patients experienced clinical relapse within 6 weeks of starting the medication, and this was independent of the use of concomitant immunosuppressive medications. However, in a recent prospective, randomized, double-blind, placebo-controlled trial of 222 UC patients in remission and on maintenance UC therapy, Sandborn et al found that short-term (2 weeks) use of a celecoxib 200 mg bid (twice a day) was not associated with clinical relapse.[4] El Miedany et al similarly conducted a randomized placebo-controlled study of IBD patients in remission who were referred to a rheumatologist for the treatment of arthritis, arthralgias, and soft tissue rheumatism.[5] After 3 months of treatment with etoricoxib, 10.5% of the study group and 11.4% of the control group reported disease flare, requiring discontinuation of the medication.

The absence of large, long-term, controlled, prospective trials makes it difficult to draw definitive conclusions regarding the use of NSAIDs in IBD. There does now seem to be a preponderance of evidence that conventional NSAIDs can elicit relapse of IBD in up to one-fourth of patients, and should therefore be avoided if possible in patients with IBD, independent of whether they are on maintenance therapy.

Unless there is a contraindication, acetaminophen should always be used as a first-line agent to control arthralgias. In a patient who is already on a 5-aminosalicyclic acid

(5-ASA) drug, changing the formulation to sulfasalazine may provide additional relief. Alternatively, if acetaminophen is ineffective and the patient is not on a 5-ASA drug, then sulfasalazine can be initiated. If acetaminophen and sulfasalazine prove ineffective, we will often prescribe a trial of tramadol followed by a COX-2 inhibitor. As with any decision in medical management, informing the patient of the small but possible risk of IBD relapse following the use of a coxib is critical. As noted above, some studies suggest that COX-2 inhibitors increase the risk of an IBD flare, and the studies demonstrating the safety profiles of COX-2 inhibitors have been short-term and in patients in remission on maintenance. We recommend that the lowest dose of a selective NSAID be used for the shortest duration of time, and we prefer that the patient be on maintenance therapy for their IBD and in remission. Of course, if the patient does flare, the COX-2 inhibitor should be discontinued immediately.

It should be noted that, depending on the severity of the arthralgias, one may not be able to avoid the use of conventional NSAIDs. As with any other drug, the risk-benefit ratio of symptom management versus an IBD flare should be discussed with the patient before initiating therapy. Even in the most recent studies, there is still a greater than 70% chance that patients will tolerate NSAIDs in the short-term.[2]

Although the primary question is the treatment of IBD-associated arthralgias, the possibility that joint pains in an IBD patient could reflect underlying arthritis should always be considered since treatment in that situation should be focused on treating the underlying IBD.

References

1. Bonner GF, Fakhri A, Vennamaneni SR. A long-term cohort study of nonsteroidal anti-inflammatory drug use and disease activity in outpatients with inflammatory bowel disease. *Inflamm Bowel Dis*. 2004;10(6):751-757.

2. Takeuchi K, Smale S, Premchand P, et al. Prevalence and mechanism of nonsteroidal anti-inflammatory drug-induced clinical relapse in patients with inflammatory bowel disease. *Clin Gastroenterol Hepatol*. 2006;4(2):196-202.

3. Matuk R, Crawford J, Abreu MT, Targan SR, Vasiliauskas EA, Papadakis KA. The spectrum of gastrointestinal toxicity and effect on disease activity of selective cyclooxygenase-2 inhibitors in patients with inflammatory bowel disease. *Inflamm Bowel Dis*. 2004;10(4):352-356.

4. Sandborn WJ, Stenson WF, Brynskov J, et al. Safety of celecoxib in patients with ulcerative colitis in remission: a randomized, placebo-controlled, pilot study. *Clin Gastroenterol Hepatol*. 2006;4(2):203-211.

5. El Miedany Y, Youssef S, Ahmed I, El Gaafary M. The gastrointestinal safety and effect on disease activity of etoricoxib, a selective cox-2 inhibitor in inflammatory bowel diseases. *Am J Gastroenterol*. 2006;101(2):311-317.

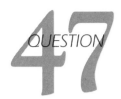

47

MY PATIENT HAS A HISTORY OF BREAST CANCER AND IS IN REMISSION FROM THAT CONDITION. SHE ALSO HAS CROHN'S DISEASE. CAN I USE AZATHIOPRINE OR INFLIXIMAB TO TREAT HER?

Remo Panaccione, MD, FRCPC

The use of immunosuppressants such as purine anti-metabolites (azathioprine, 6-mercaptopurine [6-MP], and methotrexate [MTX]) and anti-tumor necrosis factor (TNF) agents (infliximab, adalimumab, and certolizumab pegol) in patients with a previous history of solid organ malignancy and haematological malignancies is a common question that raises some controversy.

Both the purine anti-metabolites and MTX have been associated with the development of solid organ malignancies. However, one needs to look at the literature in a critical fashion before assuming this association is a contraindication for using these medications to treat someone with inflammatory bowel disease (IBD). The risk of developing solid organ malignancy seems to be more prominent in the post-transplant population, which is receiving muti-modal immunosuppressant therapy. In general, the literature does not consistently support the development of solid organ malignancies in patients who use azathioprine or 6-MP for autoimmune or inflammatory diseases.[1] There are several special circumstances that do require attention. The first is that there does appear to be an increased risk of developing non-melanotic skin cancers (basal cell carcinoma and squamous cell carcinoma) on purine anti-metabolites alone.[2] Therefore, in patients with IBD who develop non-melanotic skin cancers, I stop these agents and consider alternative therapy. The second consideration is in women who are being treated with purine anti-metabolites who appear to have a higher risk of developing cervical dysplasia.[3] I recommend that all women consider vaccination with the human papillomavirus (HPV) vaccine as outlined by the American College of Obstetrics and Gynecology screening guidelines for immunocompromised individuals. There may be an increased risk in patients who have persistent leukopenia, and, therefore, I recommend that patients on these agents be maintained within the normal range.[4] Azathioprine and 6-MP have been associated with an increased risk of developing haematological malignancies both in IBD and non-IBD patients. There does appear to be an increased risk in the development of lymphoma in patients treated with the purine anti-metabolites.[5]

The development of lymphomas is an important issue given the immunosuppressive nature of the TNF-alpha (α) inhibitors. Most lymphomas associated with TNF-α inhibitors are non-Hodgkin's lymphomas (NHL) with a mean time to onset of 10 to 21 months.[6] Post-marketing reports of lymphomas with TNF-α inhibitors have reported rates of about 0.02 to 0.03 events per 100 patient-years (expected rate in a normal population aged 65 within the SEER [Surveillance Epidemiology and End Results] database is 0.07 events per 100 patient-years). Across indications, the incidence of lymphoma in clinical trials has been estimated to be 0.11 cases per 100 patient-years (versus zero cases in placebo-treated patients).[6] The overall cancer rate in infliximab treatment arms in clinical trials is estimated to be 0.65 cases per 100 patient-years. This was 5-fold greater than placebo-treated patients, but similar to the general population rate. The incidence of lymphoma in rheumatoid arthritis (RA) patients receiving adalimumab in clinical trials has been estimated to be 0.12 cases per 100 patient-years.[6] It is important to point out that this risk estimate is similar to the background risk in the RA patient population. In the only IBD population-based study examining the incidence of lymphoma in infliximab-treated patients, an estimated annual incidence of NHL was 1.5 percent (3 patients).[7] The lymphoma was fatal in 2 patients. Approximately one-third of the patients were also receiving concomitant treatment with azathioprine. The background rate of NHL in the study population was 0.015%.

The TREAT (Crohn's Therapy Resource, Evaluation, and Assessment Tool) registry, funded by Centocor, has demonstrated similar odds of developing any cancer or lymphoma between patients receiving infliximab and patients not receiving infliximab.[8] The odds ratio (OR) for any malignancy in patients receiving infliximab compared to patients not receiving infliximab was 0.82 (95% CI, 0.48 to 1.41), and it was 1.09 (95% CI, 0.24 to 4.85) for lymphoma.[8] Although other malignancies such as rectal cancer, cutaneous T-cell lymphoma, and squamous cancer have been reported in association with adalimumab and infliximab use, their incidence rates have been similar to general population rates.[9,10] A recently published systematic review and meta-analysis of clinical trials of therapy with anti-TNF agents in RA patients derived pooled OR estimates for malignancy of 3.3 (95% CI, 1.2 to 9.1).[10] A number needed to harm (NNH) of 154 (for one additional malignancy over a treatment duration of 6 to 12 months) was calculated. However, caution must be exercised when interpreting these results, as there were a number of methodological flaws, which may have biased the study's odds estimates. Even if we assume that this study is internally valid, it may not be reasonable to generalize these results to the IBD patient population as the baseline risk of certain malignancy is likely entirely different in this population. However, despite these data, most experts believe that the risk of developing solid organ malignancies with anti-TNF therapy is extremely low to the point that anti-TNF therapy is now being investigated as adjuvant therapy in many solid organ malignancies.

The bottom line is that I would treat a patient with a history of breast cancer in remission for 5 or more years with either a purine anti-metabolite or an anti-TNF agent. In those patients with a current history of malignancy or a recent history of malignancy (less than 5 years), I usually begin therapy in conjunction with the opinion of an oncologist.

References

1. Masunaga Y, Ohno K, Ogawa R, Hashiguchi M, Echizen H, Ogata H. Meta-analysis of risk of malignancy with immunosuppressive drugs in inflammatory bowel disease. *Ann Pharmacother.* 2007;41(1):21-28.
2. Austin AS, Spiller RC. Inflammatory bowel disease, azathioprine and skin cancer: case report and literature review. *Eur J Gastroenterol Hepatol.* 2001;13(2):193-194.
3. Kane S, Khatibi B, Reddy D. Higher incidence of abnormal pap smears in women with inflammatory bowel disease. *Am J Gastroenterol.* 2008;103(3):631-636.
4. Disanti W, Rajapakse RO, Korelitz BI, Panagopoulos G, Bratcher J. Incidence of neoplasms in patients who develop sustained leukopenia during or after treatment with 6-mercaptopurine for inflammatory bowel disease. *Clin Gastroenterol Hepatol.* 2006;4(8):1025-1029.
5. Kandiel A, Fraser AG, Korelitz BI, Brensinger C, Lewis JD. Increased risk of lymphoma among inflammatory bowel disease patients treated with azathioprine and 6-mercaptopurine. *Gut.* 2005;54(8):1121-1125.
6. Keystone EC, Kavanaugh AF, Sharp JT, et al. Radiographic, clinical, and functional outcomes of treatment with adalimumab (a human anti-tumor necrosis factor monoclonal antibody) in patients with active rheumatoid arthritis receiving concomitant methotrexate therapy: a randomized, placebo controlled, 52-week trial. *Arthritis Rheum.* 2004;50(5):1400-1411.
7. Ljung T, Karlen P, Schmidt D, et al. Infliximab in inflammatory bowel disease: clinical outcome in a population based cohort from Stockholm County. *Gut.* 2004;53(6):849-853.
8. Lichenstein GR, Cohen RD, Feagan BG, et al. Safety of infliximab and other Crohn's disease therapies—TREAT registry data with nearly 15,000 patient-years of follow-up. *Gastroenterology.* 2006;130(4)(suppl 2):A71.
9. Adams AE, Zwicker J, Curiel C, et al. Aggressive cutaneous T-cell lymphomas after TNF alpha blockade. *J Am Acad Dermatol.* 2004;51(4):660-662.
10. Bongartz T, Sutton AJ, Sweeting MJ, et al. Anti-TNF antibody therapy in rheumatoid arthritis and the risk of serious infections and malignancies: systematic review and meta-analysis of rare harmful effects in randomized controlled trials. *JAMA.* 2006;295(19):2275-2285.

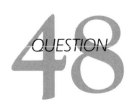

I HAVE A PATIENT WHOSE BROTHER HAS CROHN'S DISEASE. IS THERE ANYTHING I SHOULD TELL HIM TO PREVENT DISEASE ONSET OR TO DIAGNOSE THE DISEASE SOONER?

Juan L. Mendoza, MD, PhD and Maria T. Abreu, MD

There is a lot of evidence for genetic susceptibility to inflammatory bowel disease (IBD). Multiple studies have suggested that first-degree relatives of an affected patient have a risk of IBD that is 4 to 20 times as high as that among the background population. The absolute risk of IBD is approximately 7% among first-degree family members. In general, we think of Crohn's disease (CD) as more "genetic" than ulcerative colitis (UC). In CD, if you have identical twins, approximately between 50% to 58% of both twins will have CD. The risk also depends a little bit on your ethnic background. If both of your parents are Ashkenazi Jews, it raises the risk a little.[1] But beyond this fact, we know that the incidence of IBD in the Jewish population parallels the geographical diversity of the non-Jewish population of a given region. These observations hint at environmental influences.

While the exact cause of CD is unknown, there is no way to effectively prevent it (Table 48-1). Researchers believe that inherited genes, environmental factors, and the immune system all play a role (Figure 48-1). The currently accepted model of the pathogenesis of IBD is that of an inappropriate immune response to host microorganisms in genetically susceptible people. To date, no specific "trigger" has been found to cause the inflammatory response seen in CD.[2] The 2 environmental triggers we recommend avoiding in susceptible people are non-steroidal anti-inflammatory drugs (NSAIDs) and smoking. Taking aspirin, ibuprofen, or similar agents can trigger the onset of the disease, and they may be implicated in relapses of IBD. In CD, there is a 2-fold increased risk of CD in current

---

Table 48-1

Environmental Factors in Crohn's Disease Susceptibility

- Do not smoke.
- Avoid taking NSAIDs and contraceptives, except if necessary.
- Do not use antibiotics unless physician feels strongly.
- Type of diet: avoid western-type diet and increase vegetables, fruits, and fiber consumption.
- Avoid stress.
- Get regular exercise.

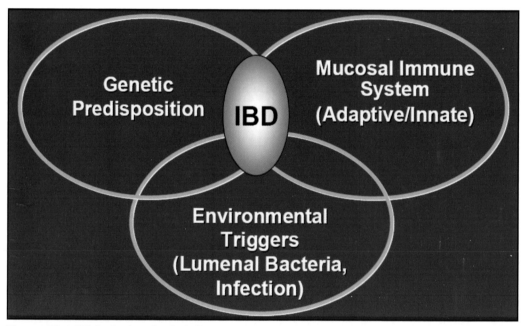

Figure 48-1. Etiologic theories in inflammatory bowel disease.

---

smokers. It turns out that things are much worse for CD patients when they smoke. They are more likely to have a flare-up, require prednisone, and require surgery. The data for passive smoking are contradictory, but most reports show that such exposure results in an increased risk of both UC and CD. Oral contraceptives have been intensively studied for a possible epidemiological or cause-and-effect relationship with IBD. The relative risk (RR) of CD in women taking oral contraceptives is about twice that of controls, although there is no direct evidence for a causative relationship. There has been controversy regarding whether women using oral contraceptives have a worse clinical outcome for IBD, but low-dose oral contraceptives do not significantly affect clinical disease activity, at least in CD. However, considering the hypercoagulability state present in active IBD, the concomitant use of oral contraceptives may aggravate the risk of thromboembolic events, but definitive data linking these factors are still lacking.

The gut bacteria have an essential role in the development of the gut immune system. The factors modifying the intestinal bacterial profile are the use of antibiotics and chemotherapeutics, the western type of diet, the modern infant nutrition, the public health measures, and the high hygienic standards and sanitation. Antibiotics can help IBD, but they can also trigger the cause. Antibiotic use has been proposed to be the central factor leading to an altered gut flora and may be the cause of dysbiosis in IBD. A fundamental dysbiosis, or imbalance between harmful and protective bacteria, has been proposed to be the root cause of IBD. Although, whether this is a primary causative factor or a secondary epiphenomenon is uncertain. This was once closely linked to diet and breastfeeding, but there is no clear evidence that either of these is a direct cause of CD. Studies seeking to link diet and IBD are generally inconclusive. Diet triggers symptoms, but occasionally, certain foods can trigger the onset of the condition. There is some evidence that a higher intake of fatty acids and frequent fast-food intake increases the risk for IBD. Trials of low carbohydrate intake have not been useful in maintaining remission or controlling flares. Anecdotal accounts of a low-fat intake being successful and pathologic demonstration of fat have led to a hypothesis that increased fats, in conjunction with bacterial antigens, play the primary role in activating the immune system and initiating CD. CD is more likely in people who eat a high-sugar, low-fiber diet. Breastfeeding confers immunity while the child's intestinal immune system is still developing. Different studies of breastfeeding and the risk of developing IBD have shown heterogeneous results, probably because of poor design. However, a subgroup analysis of high-quality studies for CD and UC have lent support to the notion that breastfeeding provides protection against IBD in offspring.

The prevalence of CD is higher in urban areas of developed countries. The traditional low incidence of IBD in developing countries, which is now on the rise, might be related to socioeconomic changes affecting hygiene. Perhaps this is because vaccination, sanitation, and sterilized foods might limit exposure to environmental antigens and impair the functional maturation of the mucosal immune system and induction of immune tolerance, which ultimately result in inappropriate immune responses when re-exposed to these antigens later in life. Stress has an impact on all medical conditions, especially cardiac disease, many gastrointestinal (GI) conditions, irritable bowel syndrome (IBS), and also IBD. The relationship between psychological stress, depression, and CD exacerbation has been controversial. However, report symptom exacerbations related to stressful life events often. New experimental evidence suggests involving direct interactions of the nervous, endocrine factors, and immune systems.

How do we make the diagnosis sooner? It is important that a careful history be taken. A physical exam will help us, but it is often nonspecific. Though CD can occur at any age, most people are diagnosed with CD between the ages of 15 and 35. Numerically, more cases are sporadic. The most common symptoms of CD are abdominal pain, often in the lower right area, and diarrhea. Rectal bleeding, black or blood in the stool, diarrhea, fever, loss of appetite, and weight loss may also occur. Laboratory tests may be helpful, and there are tests checking for anaemia, elevated white count, or C-reactive protein (CRP) and erythrocyte sedimentation rates (ESR). However, these tests in asymptomatic persons are limited by low sensitivity and specificity. By testing a stool sample, we can know if there is bleeding or infection in the intestines. We are often faced with the diagnostic difficulty of differentiating patients with IBS from those with organic intestinal pathology (in particular, IBD). Many symptoms are common to both conditions. Although symptoms are a surprisingly good guide to a diagnosis, most clinicians proceed to and rely on laboratory tests to aid in the differential diagnosis. Certainly, fulfilling the ROME criteria, and having a normal, full blood count, routine biochemical screening, ESR, and CRP are reassuring indicators pointing to IBS. The colonoscopy, small bowel X-ray, and computerized tomography are indicated for evaluation when noninvasive tests do not reveal a cause, or when inflammatory symptoms or signs are present and it is necessary to exclude all organic disease. If these diagnostic tests are negative but your patient has signs and symptoms that suggest CD, you may perform capsule endoscopy.

Screening a general population for a certain defect is useful when the sensitivity is high enough and when preventive strategies (to slow down the onset of the disease or even prevent it) are available. The fecal calprotectin test has been examined in apparently healthy first-degree relatives of patients with CD. Almost one-half of relatives had elevated fecal calprotectin concentrations, but not all subjects with high levels will progress to clinically apparent IBD. The use of fecal markers in the detection of subclinical intestinal inflammation may help in IBD, but more studies are needed. The clinical value of serological test (anti-*Saccharomyces cerevisiae* antibodies [ASCA], anti-neutrophil cytoplasmic antibodies [ANCA], and outer membrane porin protein C [OMPc]) in asymptomatic persons or in patients presenting with nonspecific GI symptoms is limited because of inadequate specificity. Recently, a study has shown that ASCA in a high-risk healthy individual might be a marker for the future development of CD, and a similar association may exist for ANCA and UC.[3] At present, the genetic testing (NOD2/CARD15) will not help distinguish CD from patients without IBD or patients with UC.[1] The other reason that this is not that helpful is that we would not know what do with the information because we could not prevent the disease. Hence, the absence of a mutation in an unaffected individual would not exclude the development of the disease, nor would the presence of a mutation necessarily lead to clinical symptoms. The RR to develop the disease when carrying at least one NOD2/CARD15 mutation is 2 to 3, but it increases dramatically to 20 to 40 in cases of 2 mutations. Recently, novel susceptibility genes have been described. Ideally, the next step should be to combine all of the available genetic markers to determinate a sooner diagnosis. For the moment, fecal, serological, and genetic tests are not worth checking as screening tests in apparently healthy first-degree relatives of patients with CD.

References

1. Van Limbergen J, Russell RK, Nimmo ER, et al. Genetics of the innate immune response in inflammatory bowel disease. *Inflamm Bowel Dis*. 2007;13(3):338-355.
2. Baumgart DC, Carding SR. Inflammatory bowel disease: cause and immunobiology. *Lancet*. 2007;369(9573): 1627-1640.
3. Israeli E, Grotto I, Gilburd B, et al. Anti-Saccharomyces cerevisiae and antineutrophil cytoplasmic antibodies as predictors of inflammatory bowel disease. *Gut*. 2005;54(9):1232-1236.

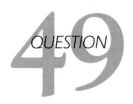

IS THE DIAGNOSIS, TREATMENT, AND RESPONSE TO TREATMENT DIFFERENT IN NONWHITES?

Robert Burakoff, MD, MPH, FACG, FACP

My initial response to the question posed above is "maybe," though this response may seem unsatisfactory to the readers of this book. The preponderance of the information we have to date is rather limited and does not allow one to draw definitive, statistically sound conclusions. However, with that being said, I will review the literature we do have available and discuss my own opinions regarding the question posed.

It is important to note that more recent epidemiological data has confirmed that the incidence and prevalence of IBD has been increasing in the African American population. In a study involving patients from northern California in the 1990's, the prevalence of IBD in the white population was 43.6/100,000 and was 29.8/100,000 for the African American population.

Most studies have confirmed that disease severity and disease behavior (ie, obstructing, inflammatory, or perforating) is similar in the African American and white populations. However, some studies have noted that the African American and Hispanic populations are more likely to have ileo-colonic or colonic disease versus ileal disease compared to the white population. This is not surprising as African Americans as well as Hispanics have significantly lower NOD2/CARD15 mutations (13%) compared to whites (40%), which is highly associated with ileal disease.[1]

The most comprehensive and largest study to date characterizing racial differences in disease phenotype in African Americans, Hispanics, and non-Hispanic whites included 830 non-Hispanic whites, 127 African Americans, and 169 Hispanics.[2] It was observed that African Americans with CD were more likely to have colorectal disease and less likely to have ileal disease, as observed in other studies. Interestingly, it was also noted that African Americans were more likely to have esophagogastroduodenal CD and perianal disease. African Americans were also at an increased risk for uveitis and sacroiliitis. Hispanics had a higher incidence of perianal disease and erythema nodosum than non-Hispanic whites, as well as more extensive colonic disease than the other groups.

It was originally proposed that African Americans had a higher incidence of perianal fistulizing disease, but a study undertaken by my IBD group in Washington, DC, in a retrospective review of 112 African Americans with CD, revealed a similar incidence compared to whites. More importantly, African Americans were more likely to have multiple fistulae and, as a result, multiple operations.[3]

Despite similarities in disease presentation and the course of the disease, quality of life questionnaires have revealed that African Americans had a lower quality of life as well as more days lost from work.[1] In addition, they were less likely to have health insurance and had difficulty getting to the doctor's appointment. Therefore, one might surmise that the diagnosis and eventual treatment might be compromised or inferior in African Americans compared to the white population because of health insurance and access issues. However, in one study, a questionnaire was administered to 148 patients with IBD—40% were white, 37% were African American, and 20% were Mexican American. All of the groups were equally likely to have regular physician visits and care given by gastroenterologists, as well as surveillance colonoscopy. Therefore, from the very limited data published, once nonwhites are in the health care system, diagnosis, treatments, and care may be similar.

There is a paucity of information on medical therapy related to the patterns of drug usage and response rates in African Americans compared to whites. In one study, there was no difference in the usage of 5-aminosalicylate (5-ASA) drugs, corticosteroids, or immunomodulatory agents. However, more recent studies cast doubt on these earlier observations. In a study at the University of Maryland of 406 patients with 102 African Americans, it was observed that African Americans received steroids, 6-mercaptopurine (6-MP)/azathroprine, and infliximab less frequently than whites.[4] Even after adjusting for disease severity, African American patients were less likely to receive 6-MP/azathroprine or infliximab. The study did not address the reasons for these differences, but one potential explanation is that African Americans have less severe disease than whites. However, there is no data (that has been published) indicating a difference in severity of disease between whites and nonwhites. If African Americans are not receiving immunomodulatory therapy as frequently as whites, other possible explanations include the high risk of being uninsured, having less access to healthcare, and the underutilization of the care offered by Medicare and Medicaid. Furthermore, minorities have greater satisfaction when seeing a provider of the same race, which results in race discordant relationships.

Is there a difference among whites, African Americans, and Hispanics undergoing surgery? The best study we have to date is from the discharge records of the Nationwide Inpatient Sample.[5] 23,389 discharges with the diagnosis of ulcerative colitis (UC) from 1998-2003 were analyzed for colectomy rates among non-Hispanic whites, African Americans, and Hispanics. The data revealed that colectomy rates were lower for African Americans and Hispanics compared to whites. Furthermore, compared to whites, African Americans had a longer interval from the time of admission to colectomy. There are several "possible" explanations for these significant observations. These include a possible higher threshold for surgery, either by choice of the patient or physician decision, and decreased access to colorectal surgeons who can perform ileal pouch-anal anastomosis (IPAA) procedures, especially in rural areas. Interestingly, patients with Medicare insurance had lower rates of colectomy. It is important to note that during this 6-year period, the rate of colectomy was decreasing for whites, but not for African Americans or Hispanics. This could indicate that African Americans and Hispanics have less access to the more expensive biological medical therapies. Since minorities comprise no more than 5% of multi-centered clinical trials for medical therapy, it is impossible to draw any conclusions regarding long-term response to medical therapies, especially the newer biological treatments, including anti-tumor necrosis factor (TNF) therapies. So what can we conclude from the review of the literature above? I will summarize my personal observations and possible conclusions drawn from the limited information we have.

We have no data that the initial diagnostic approach to IBD in nonwhites is any different than in whites. There is emerging data that nonwhites may not always be receiving optimal medical therapy, more likely as a result of being underinsured and having less access to care. There is no data indicating a difference in response to medical therapy for nonwhites versus whites.

My experience has been that nonwhites respond similarly to 5-ASA, corticosteroids, and immunomodulatory therapy, including biological therapies. I have also noted that surgery is performed in a timely manner, regardless of race or ethnic background. It is disturbing to note the limited literature we have indicates a delay in surgery, varying geographically, in nonwhites versus whites. This observation must be confirmed within prospective studies. We have no data on postsurgical recurrence rates in nonwhites versus whites. Further studies are needed to follow the long-term postsurgical outcomes of nonwhites versus whites to determine response to medical therapy when indicated. Additionally, we need to study the frequency of colon cancer screening and the risk of colon cancer in IBD in the nonwhite population.

Finally, with the increasing prevalence of IBD in the nonwhite population, it is of utmost importance that we make every effort to include significantly more nonwhites in multi-centered clinical trials to determine the best treatment regimens.

References

1. Jackson JF, Kornbluth A. Do black and Hispanic Americans with inflammatory bowel disease (IBD) receive inferior care compared with white Americans? *Am J Gastroenterol.* 2007;102(7):1343-1349.
2. Nguyen GC, Torres EA, Regueiro M, et al. Inflammatory bowel disease characteristics among African Americans, Hispanics, and non-Hispanics whites: characterization of a large North American cohort. *Am J Gastroenterol.* 2006;101(5):1012-1023.
3. Reddy SI, Burakoff R. Inflammatory bowel disease in African Americans. *Inflamm Bowel Dis.* 2003;9(6):380-385.
4. Flasar MH, Johnson T, Roghmann M, Cross RK. Disparities in the use of immunomodulators and biologics for the treatment of inflammatory bowel disease: a retrospective cohort study. *Inflamm Bowel Dis.* 2008;14(1):13-19.
5. Nguyen GC, Laveist TA, Gearhart S, et al. Racial and geographic variations in colectomy rates among hospitalized ulcerative colitis patients. *Clin Gastroenterol Hepatol.* 2006;4(12):1507-1513.

INDEX

CURBSIDE
Consultation

The exciting and unique *Curbside Consultation Series* is designed to effectively provide gastroenterologists with practical, to the point, evidence based answers to the questions most frequently asked during informal consultations between colleagues.

Each specialized book included in the *Curbside Consultation Series* offers quick access to current medical information with the ease and convenience of a conversation. Expert consultants who are recognized leaders in their fields provide their advice, preferences, and solutions to 49 of the most frequent clinical dilemmas in gastroenterology.

Written with a similar reader-friendly Q and A format and including images, diagrams, and references, each book in the *Curbside Consultation Series* will serve as a solid, go-to reference for practicing gastroenterologists and residents alike.

Series Editor: Francis A. Farraye, MD, MSc, FACP, FACG

Curbside Consultation in Endoscopy:
49 Clinical Questions
Joseph Leung, MD; Simon Lo, MD
250 pp., Soft Cover, 2009,
ISBN 978-1-55642-817-3,
Order #78170, **$79.95**

Curbside Consultation of the Colon:
49 Clinical Questions
Brooks D. Cash, MD, FACP, CDR, MC, USN
208 pp., Soft Cover, 2009,
ISBN 978-1-55642-831-9,
Order #78316, **$79.95**

Curbside Consultation in GERD:
49 Clinical Questions
Philip Katz, MD
192 pp., Soft Cover, 2008,
ISBN 978-1-55642-818-0,
Order #78189, **$79.95**

Curbside Consultation of the Liver:
49 Clinical Questions
Mitchell Shiffman, MD
272 pp., Soft Cover, 2008,
ISBN 978-1-55642-815-9,
Order #78154, **$79.95**

Curbside Consultation in IBD:
49 Clinical Questions
David Rubin, MD; Sonia Friedman, MD;
Francis A. Farraye, MD
240 pp., Soft Cover, 2009,
ISBN 978-1-55642-856-2,
Order #78562, **$79.95**

Curbside Consultation of the Pancreas:
49 Clinical Questions
Scott Tenner, MD, MPH;
Alphonso Brown MD, MS Clin Epi
250 pp., Soft Cover, 2009,
ISBN 978-1-55642-814-2,
Order #78146, **$79.95**

WWW.CURBSIDECONSULTATIONS.COM